Living

Less Toxic

BY THE SAME AUTHOR

CLEANSE

LOVING YOURSELF INSIDE AND OUT

Living a Life Less Toxic

FAITH CANTER

EMPOWERED
BOOKS

Published in 2018 by Empowered Books

Copyright © Faith Canter 2018
2nd edition
Originally published by Balboa Press in 2015

Faith Canter has asserted her right to be identified as the author of this
Work in accordance with the Copyright, Designs and Patents Act 1988

ISBN Paperback: 978-0-9957047-4-9
Ebook: 978-0-9957047-5-6

A CIP catalogue copy of this book can be found in the British Library.

Published with the help of Indie Authors World
indieauthorsworld.com

IndieAuthors
World

DEDICATION

To one of life's true legends...

A man who's always believed in, supported, listened to and loved me, no matter what nonsense I am up to, who I am with, or where I am in the world:

Happy 80th Birthday Year Les, you really are one in a million!

I feel truly blessed to have you in my life, to call you my step-dad and to have shared so many special memories with you.

You have always inspired me with your positivity, strength, energy, determination and authenticity. You give selflessly, care compassionately and show us all how to enjoy the simple pleasures of life, with laughter, honesty and passion.

If everyone could have a Les in their life, their lives would be all the richer for it!

Thank you for coming into my life, for showing me there is another way to be a human being and for being you, Les.

Faith xx

CONTENTS

Why Did I Write This Book?   11

Introduction   15

Present Moment Awareness   19

Breath   35

The Attitude of Gratitude   45

Self-talk and Self-love   53

Less Toxic Thoughts   63

Less Toxic Bodies   77

Foodie Facts   87

Digestive Health   97

Favourite Raw Food Recipes   102

The Little Critters   161

Does Eating Organic Really Make a Difference?   169

Healthy Recipes   175

    Breakfast Recipes   176

    Lunch Recipes   189

    Dinner Recipes   208

    Snack Recipes   233

    Side Dishes Recipes   238

    Desserts   248

A Less Toxic Home   263

Less Toxic Body Care Products   269

    Household Product Recipes   279

Less Toxic Homecare Products   305

    Home Care Product Recipes   307

Detoxing our Four-Legged Friends   317

De-Junking Home, Health & Office   329

Nature Nurtures   343

When Being Less Toxic Becomes Toxic!   353

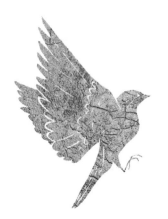

WHY DID I WRITE THIS BOOK?

I'm Scottish-born, but was raised in the south of England. Although thoroughly loved by my family, I grew to be deeply unhappy with myself and my life. I was abused as a small child and then allowed myself to be used by many as I grew up. I thought if I could be who I thought people wanted me to be, then I would make them happy, make them love me and I would be happy then too. I tried to be the helper, the pleaser, the achiever and the perfectionist; I was unsuccessful at all. I was desperate for attention and love, and sought it out in all the wrong places. My depression and self-loathing spiralled out of control and I only felt happy when taking drugs or drinking. I regularly cut myself, suffered from eating disorders and more, and all too often fantasised about leaving my miserable life.

In my late teens I became quite unwell, suffering from insomnia, OCDs, Irritable Bowel Syndrome (IBS), food intolerances, headaches, fatigue and depression.

Eventually, some years later, I caught a very bad stomach bug in India that lasted for months. On returning to the UK, I contracted glandular fever, which then turned into Myalgic Encephalopathy / Chronic Fatigue Syndrome (ME/CFS). I learnt later that I had been wandering around with adrenal fatigue for many years prior to getting ME/CFS and so had nothing left to fight it with.

Today, I have not only recovered from ME/CFS, but I have also recovered from all the other illnesses and feel a strength both mentally and physically that I never felt possible before.

The contents of this book are what assisted my recovery from all my mental and physical health ailments, and how I finally stopped fighting myself and my life. It's how I found my happy and healthy place in life, and all this was done from detoxing mind, body and environment.

Some time after writing the first edition of this book, I realised I had missed out some important stuff! And my perspective on a few things shifted had throughout the lengthy publication process, and a lot since then too. You'll notice I talk about the importance of self-love, simplifying life, and when being less toxic can become toxic. These topics come up daily with my coaching clients and within workshops and training sessions, so they deserve a proper mention here. Not only this, but you'll see that pushing on through is usually not the best course of action when trying to heal, find happiness and live harmoniously in this crazy-ass world. Instead, listening to ourselves, making friends with who we are and living compassionately and honestly, is.

I wanted to share with you what has helped me, because I hope some of what I share helps you to see you are not alone, you can get through this, and just because living toxically seems to be the norm in modern society, it does not have to be the norm for *you and your family!*

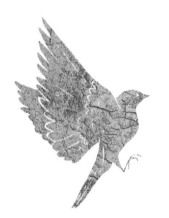

INTRODUCTION

If you are sick and tired of feeling sick and tired, then you are in the right place!

When clients come to see me, they are often at the end of their tether. They have often spent a considerable sum of money trying to 'fix' themselves, or they believe that they don't have the ability, funds or time to make the changes they feel they need to make. Quite often they have addressed one part of their health, but not the others. Could this be you, too? This book teaches you a whole-life approach to health and well-being. It discusses practical, easy, cheap and, in many instances, time-saving methods for making enjoyable and healthy changes to your lifestyle. These small changes can have a huge positive impact on how you feel, think, see yourself, others, and your environment.

Living a Life Less Toxic is about reducing the toxic load of your mind, body, home and environment, without reducing your bank balance or your quality of life. This approach to reducing toxins from every level of your life is a clear-cut way to a happier and healthier future.

Many more of us are no longer happy to accept the use and application of toxic chemicals or products just because they are cheap and easily accessible. We are realising that we need to take the bull by the horns and be the masters of our own health and well-being. We are becoming more aware of what living in the 21st century is doing to our own health and that of our planet. We are slowly taking back control and saying no to things we do not like. Just because it has become the norm to smother ourselves in toxic chemicals and live in toxic homes, it does not have to be *your* norm! You can choose another way, and I hope the words and recipes shared within these pages show you it's not as hard as it may seem.

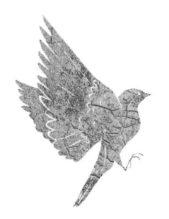

CHAPTER 1

PRESENT MOMENT AWARENESS

If you can resist the impulse to claim each and every thought as your own, you will come to a startling conclusion: you will discover that you are the consciousness in which the thoughts appear and disappear –
Annamalai Swami

Our minds are amazing, complicated and computer-like and we simply don't give them enough credit. Instead, we often do the complete opposite and put them under immense and continued pressure. We also allow our minds to run away with themselves, generating problems, plans, concepts, running over old ground again and again, getting sucked into stories and worrying about the future and what could, (but will most likely not), be!

I don't know about you, but over the years I've found this whole daily routine completely exhausting. Constantly second-guessing people, events, being paranoid, and worrying about things that will probably never happen. I've had many sleepless nights, due to a head full of craziness like this. All this is good for is making us tired, grumpy and if you're really unlucky, ill!

If we could just show our crazy brains how to be more present, we'd find more peace, happiness, fulfilment and health. Our mind just needs to be reminded how to become the observer, not part of the current of the *what has beens, what could bes and what never will bes.*

Our minds are still pre-programmed with the fight or flight response from many, many generations ago. It's the same response that animals have to help them deal with danger. As soon as they notice something that they perceive to be a threat, they instantly go into fight or flight mode. This response gives them a surge of adrenaline to enable them to run from or fight their potential attacker. We humans still have this response within us. However, these days, we don't need to fight a dinosaur or a sabre-toothed tiger. In the modern world, our fight or flight response kicks in when we feel threatened or stressed in other ways. This could be due to work commitments, family issues, relationships, health concerns, concerns for loved ones, or for many of us, all of the above! So, although we may joke that our boss is a dinosaur, actually our brain may be reacting as if they actually are.

It's normal to worry, dwell on events and plans - that's part of what makes us human. However, when we constantly do this, then our minds and bodies start to think we need the fight or flight response. That's when our bodies start to produce more adrenaline.

Adrenaline and cortisol (the steroid hormone that the adrenal glands produce when we require an additional burst of hormones) hamper our sleep, make us feel edgy, stressed, and unable to deal with normal day-to-day things. The longer this goes on, the longer the body feels it's under attack. It tries to support us with more hormones, which when produced long-term, create more health issues, including digestive problems, fatigue, weight gain, hair loss, emotional instability, and more. You may or may not recognise some of this, but it's what we generally refer to as chronic stress!

Our amazing bodies simply cannot cope with long-term stress; they cannot continue to maintain the levels of the hormones produced when we are in this long-term fight or flight response.

I know this all too well. Unknowingly, I had been suffering from adrenal fatigue for many years. I was a worrier, an over-thinker, a past trauma re-player and an over-planner. I barely slept, ate mostly the wrong foods, and burnt the candle at both ends. I was young, and this is what I thought young people did. Right? Wrong!

One day, along came glandular fever. My body had nothing left to fight with, and I had a chronic condition that stayed with me for over six years - Chronic Fatigue Syndrome / Myalgic Encephalomyelitis (ME). My story isn't unique. I have worked with hundreds of clients, all with very similar stories to mine.

I would like you to understand that the level of stress we put ourselves under these days is not normal - just because everyone is feeling it, it doesn't mean we can maintain it. Therefore, it often leads to health issues if not addressed.

During my years of ill health, I tried many different approaches, pills, potions and various other medical suggestions. None of this worked for me. In fact, I ended up with more symptoms than I'd started with, and, added to those were the side-effects from medications.

No one ever asked me about my mental state of mind, my history or my stress levels. No one asked me if I had any symptoms prior to CFS/ME. I did have symptoms, but I'd put them down to the result of burning the candle at both ends and the belief that no one I knew seemed to have perfect health. I also noticed that, no matter how much sleep or rest I got, I was always tired. My body would rest, but my mind never could. I was worrying about my health as well as everything else I was dwelling on. I was getting worse!

I had enough. I started to do my own research, and I found a trend in all of us worriers, over-thinkers, doers, planners, trauma re-players: *it was adrenal fatigue.* It seems I'd had it for many years. I knew that I had to do something to change things, come hell or high water.

I realised that I had to bring my stress and anxiety levels down. This was a little unnerving for me as I'd always thought I worked best under pressure. It's possible this was the case when dealing with a pile of papers on my desk, but it simply wasn't good for my mental and physical health. Nor was it for my co-workers!

Mindfulness and Meditation

Time and time again, I came across articles, books, and research about the merits of meditation for all sorts of health concerns, but especially for stress-related issues. I thought, 'There's no way I can quieten my mind, there's no way I can even sit for that long, let alone meditate.' But there was also no way I wanted to continue to feel so awful, day in, day out. So, even though I had had absolutely no previous experience of it, or even really knew what I was doing, I started daily guided meditations. Within a few days, I'd gone from having less than four hours' broken sleep a night to eight hours' solid sleep, and this has continued (if I continue the meditation) for most nights ever since.

I chose guided meditation at the beginning, as, like many others, I'd had no luck with the silent, self-guided kind. This was because I incorrectly assumed that silent meditation was all about making the mind go blank, quiet, and clear. Being quiet just made me think, plan and plot even more. I didn't realise at the time that this is not what silent meditations are all about.

I found this quote among my Mindfulness training paperwork (from the Mindfulness Association) that beautifully explains what meditation is really all about, and I thought it might be helpful to share it here:

Mindfulness analogy of undercurrent and observer

A useful analogy for explaining the undercurrent and observer is someone sitting on the bank of a river and watching the water flow by. The river is like the undercurrent and the observer is the one who sits on the bank. Sometimes the river is turbulent and other times it flows smoothly; sometimes it washes logs and debris downstream, whilst other times the water is clear and translucent. Our minds are like this. The key instruction in mindfulness practice is to remain sitting on the bank of the river, watching the changing flow.

The various mindfulness methods are ways of assisting us in remaining grounded in this observing mode, and staying on the bank. When we become distracted and involved with what is flowing by, it is like jumping into the river and being carried along in its flow, sometimes tumbling over waterfalls, other times getting caught amongst the swirling debris, while other times basking in a still, clear pool.

The key point is that we are caught in the flow and vulnerable to where it takes us, sometimes in a desirable direction, while other times in the direction of confusion and suffering. What pulls us into the river are the likes and dislikes of the observer - the one sitting on the bank. We like some things and grasp at them and we dislike other things and push them away. Either way we fall in.

I always recommend guided meditation to beginners, because having someone guide you through a meditation, even if it's a recording, helps keep you grounded and your mind from following your own random thoughts. I still like to use guided meditations myself from time to time, as they keep things fresh.

So how does this amazing tool work?

When we meditate, we bring our mind into the present moment. We stop focusing on the past, the future, the worries, the plans and all those other people. Instead, we focus on whatever the meditation is about or simply remember to let the thoughts float right on by.

During this time, our mind stops being busy, it rests and recuperates and our body starts to repair and rejuvenate (just like while sleeping). This in turn reduces the 'fight or flight' response, and our anxiety and stress levels begin to subside.

If you meditate daily, regularly giving your mind that quiet time, the body starts to repair itself from the years of being in the stress cycle: the benefits of this can be huge. These are some of them:

Meditation:

- ❀ reduces stress, anxiety and panic attacks

- ❀ enhances the immune system

- ❀ increases blood flow through the body

- ❀ lowers blood pressure

- ❀ reduces headaches and migraines

- ❀ increases mental clarity

- ❀ increases stamina

- ❀ balances hormones

- ❀ improves the flow of air in the lungs

- ❀ reduces insomnia

- ❀ helps you feel grounded

- ❀ reduces aggression

- ❀ helps with addictions

- ❀ reduces pain in the body

- ❀ releases tension from the body.

Any meditation is better than no meditation, so if you really can only make time for three minutes of meditation a day, then just do three minutes. Even this small amount of time each day can lead to more productivity, focus, energy and clarity, meaning you'll get back the time 'lost' in each meditation tenfold. Really!

Below is a short meditation transcript for beginners. You can make a recording of this meditation yourself to play it back, or you can visit my YouTube channel to listen to the meditation for free on my meditation playlist there.

The important thing with all meditations is to find a comfortable position. Don't get too hung up on having to sit a certain way on a meditation stool or a cushion. Simply find a spot where you will not be disturbed, switch off phones, computers and other distractions and make sure you are comfortable and at the right temperature.

When I first started, I wasn't well enough to be able to sit for the length of time it took to meditate, so I used to lie down. Sometimes I'd fall asleep, but I saw that that was ok, too. Your body will do what it needs when you meditate; don't give it a hard time. If you need to sleep, allow sleep to come. If you start thinking, then do not give yourself a hard time for thinking, just observe the thoughts, rather than being consumed by them. Whatever is needed will come, and eventually, once you start to create a routine of meditating, all the benefits of it will follow.

Find a comfortable position, somewhere where you won't be disturbed, where you are warm enough, but not where it's too hot or stuffy. Make sure your position is well-supported.

Close your eyes.

Relax your muscles, making sure your face, neck, shoulders and back muscles are all relaxed.

Notice your breathing, how your breath flows in and out.

Make no effort to change your breathing in any way, simply notice how your body breathes.

When your attention wanders, (as it will), just focus again on your breathing.

Do not give yourself a hard time if your mind wanders,

simply recognise it has, and return to the breathing.

See how your breath continues to flow in and out, deeply and calmly.

Feel the air entering through your nose and filling your whole body with beautiful healing light and energy. Then notice the slight pause before it begins to leave your body through your slightly pursed lips, and again, notice a slight pause before the cycle begins once more.

Feel your chest and stomach gently rise and fall with each breath.

Notice how cleansing each breath feels and appreciate this gift you are giving to yourself.

See how calm and gentle your breathing is, and how relaxed your body feels.

Now, notice the sounds around you. Start with the sounds outside, then bring your attention to the sounds in the room, and lastly, to the sounds of your own body.

Feel the chair or the floor beneath you, how your body touches this and where.

Feel your clothes against your body.

Move your fingers and toes.

Roll your shoulders.

Open your eyes and remain sitting for a few moments longer.

Then stretch your arms and legs gently.

Sit for a few more moments, enjoying how relaxed you

feel, and thank yourself for this gift you have given yourself.

After five or ten minutes, go about your normal day, knowing you have done something fundamentally good for yourself!

Being Present

After I had begun meditating regularly, I found my anxiety and stress levels dropped a little from having more sleep and from spending a small amount of my day not hanging out in my crazy brain but meditating instead. However, I knew most of my waking hours were spent focusing on the past, the future, all the 'could bes', 'should bes' and 'bad mes'.

I knew this wasn't good for my mental health, but I was shocked to find out what an impact it was having on my physical health too. I didn't realise that all this underlying overthinking was triggering my nervous system, which in the long term, can start to affect many other systems of the body, like the digestive and endocrine systems for starters. It began to make a lot of sense to me why most of the people I knew with ME/CFS had digestive issues and/or hormonal issues too. We all think these are separate issues, but it turns out they aren't! Or at the very least, they are made much, much worse by this constant overthinking and over-analysing.

It seemed to me that being more present in as many of my daily moments as possible, not just whilst meditating, was part of the key to unlocking the crippling effects of underlying overthinking. But how? My mind did what it wanted to do, I felt I had no control over it or how it made me feel; I felt stuck!

This was when I came across *mindfulness*. It seemed too simple to work, but that's the beauty of it - it is simple and it does work!

Mindfulness is a word given to 'being present in the moment', having our awareness right here, right now, rather than in the past or the future. Often during the course of our day, we knowingly or unknowingly slip into this loop of thinking about past events and future worries. This only serves to keep us in a stress response.

But we can be present whilst walking, doing the dishes, cutting the grass, or basically anything during our day. And, the more our awareness is in the present moment, the less we are in any sort of stress response and the less anxiety and depression we are likely to suffer as a result.

How does it work?

When you become aware that your head is off worrying about the past or the future, simply breathe and come back to the moment. Look at what you are doing, really look. Notice how amazing it is to have hot water flowing from the tap, washing-up liquid to clean away the grease, food to make the dishes dirty and to nourish your body to be able to do these things. Notice your breath, your body, your surroundings, sounds around you, the weather - whatever there is to notice. Open your eyes and heart to the present moment, being fully immersed in it. Let go of it needing to be anything else than it actually is. Your mind will wander, but that's ok, just softly (without telling yourself off) bring your awareness back to the present moment once more.

The more your practice this, the easier it becomes to hang out in the present moment, and the less stressed, anxious and depressed you will feel. Not only this, but the more time spent *here* means the body also spends more time in a healing state, so it not only benefits mental health, but physical health too.

Being present while walking

I love to hike: it fills me with great joy, appreciation and a sense of freedom, and even more so since being so ill for so long. Walking is a perfect time to practice mindfulness, not just as a means of speeding from A to B. It doesn't have to be a big hike, just a walk to the shops or around the garden or even the house. Take a look at the guidance below for being more present whilst walking...

Take a few deep breaths and set the intention that during your walk, you will try to be aware of your environment and how you interact with it.

As you start to walk, notice the sensation of your feet hitting the ground with each step. How does this feel?

As you move your legs, which muscles tense or relax as you move? How does this feel?

Notice where you are stepping. Are you stepping hard or lightly onto the ground? Are you being gentle with yourself?

Expand your awareness to notice your surroundings. What do you see, smell, hear and feel?

Expand your awareness so that you remain aware of your whole environment, as well as how you fit into this environment and how you move through it.

Are thoughts crossing your mind as you walk? There's no

need to judge these internal experiences as good or bad. Practise just being an observer of them, and then draw your attention back to your awareness of the walk, and your part in it.

As you complete your walk, thank yourself for this gift.

Every day, I speak to people who have literally turned their lives around due to living more in their moments and/or enjoying meditation or similar practices. I've shared my experience with you because I wanted you to hear my story first-hand, so you can see what all this underlying overthinking can do to us and how we can fix it without pills or potions.

I tried all manner of standard medications, and none of them worked. Maybe you can relate to my story? I haven't come across one person who hasn't been helped in some way by adding meditation to their daily life. Not all forms of meditation work for everyone and certainly not in the same way. So don't give up if the first one you try doesn't work for you: there are hundreds, if not thousands of methods out there, so have fun trying them out. At the very least, this daily practice will give you some peace and space in your day for you and you alone. The possibilities are endless.

Why not give meditation a go, and see how you get on? It's an amazing way to start to notice the beautiful world around you. It opens up your eyes to things you'd usually walk straight past or wouldn't give a second glance. It helps you lose the beauty blinkers you may be wearing and assists in bringing balance back to mind, body and soul.

Resources

www.faithcanter.com/videos

Secrets of Meditation - Davidji

Mind Calm - Sandy Newbigging

Body Calm – Sandy Newbigging

The Power of Now - Eckhart Tolle

Mindfulness: A practical guide to finding peace in a frantic world - Prof. Mark Williams

Adrenal Fatigue: The 21st Century Stress Syndrome - Dr James Wilson

Is it Me or is it my Adrenals? - Marcelle Pick

The Cortisol Connection - Shawn Talbott

The Mindfulness Association -

www.mindfulnessassociation.org

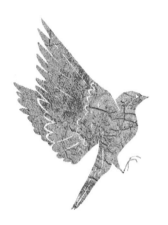

CHAPTER 2

BREATH

*Remember to breathe. It is after all, the secret of life –***Gregory Maguire**

You may be wondering why there is a chapter on breath and posture. Why wouldn't you be breathing correctly and what difference does this have to the toxic load of your body? You've been breathing all your life and you're still alive, right? In fact, it's something your body does without you even having to think about it, so what's the problem?

Obviously, we all breathe, but generally not in a very efficient way for our bodies. By this I mean that we breathe far too shallowly, and this hinders many functions in our body. Shallow breathing can create respiratory problems, anxiety and panic attacks. It can create tension throughout the body, fatigue, weakness of the body's core, and hinders the elimination of toxins. In her book *Effortless Pain Relief*, Dr Ingrid Bacci explains that shallow breathing means that we become less efficient in delivering all the oxygen required by our bodies; she also explains the health implications this can have for us.

The bottom half of the lung is around twice as effective as the top half of the lung in supplying us with our required amount of oxygen. The bottom half also expels twice as many toxins, so when we don't use the bottom half, we are making the body work harder and expelling fewer toxins.

Another common issue when we don't breathe effectively is that the old air is not expelled properly: a little fresh air is mixed with a little old air we've kept hold of. This gives our bodies just enough oxygen to function, but not much more. We need to expel almost all of the air with each breath for full bodily functioning and for optimum detoxification. A classic example of this is what happens when we are stressed, panicked, or feeling anxious. We tend to take short, shallow breaths, but if we take a big, deep breath, we take in a full lungful of air, expel all the old air, and then our stress levels begin to go down. It relaxes our muscles, calms our emotions, and heightens mental clarity. This is why we are often told to take long, deep breaths when panicked or stressed. It has a physical, as well as an emotional, healing effect on us. This is also why people who smoke believe that having a cigarette helps to de-stress and calm them down. This calming effect is actually caused by the long, deep drags on the cigarette which does include taking in air, and very little by the replenishment of the nicotine in their bodies (although feeding the addiction does help for a few seconds).

Consider these symptoms of incorrect breathing:

- ❀ increased stress and anxiety
- ❀ increased toxicity in the body
- ❀ low energy levels
- ❀ depleted brain function

- ❀ digestive issues
- ❀ light-headedness
- ❀ poor concentration
- ❀ memory loss
- ❀ numbness (hands and fingers)
- ❀ poor circulation
- ❀ coldness
- ❀ muscular spasms
- ❀ twitching
- ❀ excessive sneezing
- ❀ excessive mucus
- ❀ excessive sighing
- ❀ excessive yawning
- ❀ long-term blocked or runny sinuses
- ❀ shortness of breath
- ❀ difficulty in swallowing
- ❀ abdominal bloating
- ❀ belching and flatulence
- ❀ constant fatigue
- ❀ general weakness
- ❀ insomnia
- ❀ palpitations
- ❀ skipped heartbeats
- ❀ tachycardia

Do you recognise any of those symptoms in yourself? If so, here are some simple things you can do to help promote healthy and more effective breathing:

1. Breathe into the stomach, your back and the bottom part of the lungs, rather than just the top part of the lungs. Pay attention to these areas and fill them as full of breath as you can. Breathing into the back not only helps with physical issues, but also has the potential for psychological healing: it allows you to address things you have tried unsuccessfully to put behind you.

2. Concentrate on the physical function of breathing: observe how this feels, where you feel it, where you are breathing in and out from, and where you feel any tension. Imagine this tension leaving your body as you breathe out.

3. When you breathe in, push your stomach out, and when you breathe out, let your stomach go in. This is called 'belly breathing' and this is what most people who meditate and practice yoga do (it takes some getting used to, but it's worth it). If you look at the way a baby breathes, it is exactly like this. Somewhere along the line, we lose this natural way of breathing and replace it with its opposite.

4. A couple of times a day, breathe into the whole body, not just your core. Feel your whole body expand and become energised by this fulfilling breath.

5. Practice this one regularly: Breathe out as far as you can, hold it for a few seconds (when you hold your breath here, your body is in its optimum state of transfer between carbon dioxide and oxygen, and this is a really beneficial time to linger in, for both your body and mind). Then breathe in as far as you can and hold this for a few seconds also (again lingering in this optimum state of transfer). Repeat this a few times. This opens up your whole lung capacity and helps to eliminate as many toxins as possible from your respiratory system.

6. Imagine you are breathing out all your negativity and bad emotions and breathing in fresh, positive and healing energy and emotions. This has a dramatic positive effect on both your body and mind.

7. Do some guided breathing meditations for optimum breath work and thus health. You can find lots of these online, including on my YouTube Channel.

It's all about retraining yourself to breathe properly and to spend time each day doing these techniques so that you can establish a new, healthy habit.

Another very simple and effective way to enhance good breathing is to promote good posture. This is possibly one of the most effective tools in your correct breathing handbook!

If you are slouched over or bunched up in any way, this means the lungs, as well as other organs in the body, cannot work effectively. Just by sitting upright on a sturdy chair, you will notice that you immediately start to feel more energised and engaged. This is because the lungs can take in more oxygen, and then move this oxygen more easily around the body.

Slouching also puts the body under additional strain because muscles are being used that aren't made for supporting the body. This is why people often fall asleep when slouched on the sofa. However, you may have noticed that if you need to stay awake, you'll find you are propping yourself upright. This is a subconscious act on the part of your body to get more oxygen and thus feel more awake.

Here are some of the benefits of correct posture:

- improves quality of breathing
- improves the elimination of toxins from the body
- reduces back pain and associated issues
- reduces tension and anxiety
- improves circulation
- improves energy
- increases concentration and mental performance
- helps to prevent beer bellies (as it keeps the abdominal muscles in shape)
- helps your body become aligned
- decreases muscle and joint wear (promotes bone health)
- aids digestion

So what can you do to promote good posture?

1. Listen to your body. If you're uncomfortable, then move.

If it hurts when you sit for long periods of time, then move. If you're in pain, then move. If you work at a desk all day, then... yes you've got it, get up and move about regularly. It is really important: move about as often as possible.

2. Keep your body aligned as much as possible. That means distributing your weight evenly on/over your feet and hips when standing, and your buttocks when sitting. A tip: your ears, shoulders and hips should be in alignment whenever possible.

3. When carrying bags, make sure the weight is distributed evenly. Either use a rucksack (making sure you use both straps) or split the weight between two bags, carrying one in each hand.

4. Do not overstretch when working for prolonged periods of time at desks and benches.

5. Exercise moderately to help keep your core strong, your body healthy and supple, thus reducing the risk of injury and increasing its overall strength.

6. Flat shoes are always best! That goes for you too, gentlemen! Seriously though, we all know heels aren't good for our backs, so if you must wear them, only do it for short bursts so there's less stress on the body and most importantly, so that your posture doesn't suffer.

7. Follow your basic health and safety training, i.e. bend from the knees when lifting things, don't twist or

overstretch and don't try to lift a heavy load by yourself.

8. Lastly, try to relax: tension and anxiety in our muscles inhibits good posture.

Helpful Hints

If we remember to stop and breathe whenever we are feeling under pressure, overwhelmed, stuck, confused, angry, basically when any of our persistent negative thoughts are running the show, then we give ourselves that moment of space to come back to ourselves, to not get totally lost in the 'crazy brain show' and to understand where we are and how to move forward. This simple act of taking a breath not only assists the body in all the ways mentioned above, but it's an amazing way of bringing some respite to the mind too!

Resources

*Effortless Pain Relief - **Dr Ingrid Bacci***

www.faithcanter.com/videos

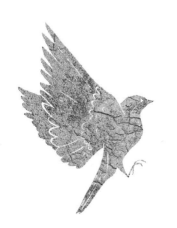

CHAPTER 3

THE ATTITUDE OF GRATITUDE

*We can complain because rose bushes have thorns, or
rejoice because thorns have roses* – **Alphonse Karr**

As I mentioned previously, we are instinctively programmed to look for potential problems. This would have been and still is, to a degree, part of how we make sure we and our loved ones are safe. We instinctively weigh up new situations, people, places and environments as we come across them, and more often than not, this saves us from bad situations.

What we need to try to do is to form new habits and new pathways in the brain, so that we can begin to instinctively look for positive things around us rather than negative. I'm not sure if you've noticed, but when you start focusing on negative things, more negative things happen, and when you start focusing on positive things, more positive things happen. That's because, whichever direction we are focusing in, we are strengthening our neural pathways within the brain. By focusing continually on the positive, we begin to build more positive, empowering pathways. In turn, these pathways enhance positive chemical processes in the brain and the body.

So how do you achieve this? You can start to train your brain to look for the positive things that happen during your daily routines rather than focusing on the negative things. Making mental and/or physical lists of the things you are grateful for, and not the things that are wrong, is a great place to start. Once you start to write these down, you form new habits and find it easier and easier to find more positive things to be grateful for. You need to get really good at retraining your mind and creating new and healthy habits. Before long, you won't even need to consciously think about it, and these thought processes will just happen of their own accord.

A Learning Curve

Whilst I was writing the first edition of this book, I launched a new site for another project I was working on to do with my recovery from ME/CFS. I shared this site on a forum that I had been a member of for some time. Within minutes I started to get feedback from people on the forum: 95% of it was really lovely, positive and encouraging, but 5% was very negative, rude, and felt like a personal attack. Can you guess (even with all the work I'd done on myself) which feedback I instantly chose to focus on? Yep, the 5%!

I became quite fixated on their remarks, brushing aside all the wonderful remarks I'd received about my new project, and I got quite upset by the whole situation. I had worked so hard on this project, was very proud of it and wanted to share it with other people. All I'd wanted to do was help other people. Why had a handful of readers chosen to be nasty and put me down? What was wrong with my project? Or even worse, what was wrong with me? I instantly reverted back to a hurt, upset and negative thinking pattern.

But then I caught myself. I decided this wasn't healthy and I had to walk away from it and take some time out. So I went to meditate, talk to my husband and had some cuddles with my dogs.

What happened next would never have happened if it hadn't been for that 5% of negativity. Over the next few days, I told family and friends how unhappy I was about the response I had received, and I had a massive influx of positive, lovely and encouraging words from them. I didn't even know that most of these people felt this way about me or my work. I really started to feel the love, and with this, I became grateful for the 5% as they had shown me something about my life I had never even realised before. They showed me how much love and positivity there was in my life through the compassionate comments of others.

I learnt so much from this, which in turn, helped me to grow a little more as a person. My point is that it's easy to slip into old negative ways of thinking, but even during those negative times, if you look and listen, you'll find positivity hiding there somewhere. Perhaps it sets you on a new path, perhaps you meet new and influential people, or you have a great example to put in your book! The saying 'every cloud has a silver lining' really is true. It might take some time to figure out what it is, but it's there.

Practise focusing on the positive in your day-to-day life, and when something bigger and trickier comes along, the process will have become second nature to you, and it just won't seem so big or tricky.

*

Another powerful lesson in gratitude

As a child, I had been taught all about nature, the planet, and our environment. But somewhere along the line I'd lost my connection with it, or should I say I'd just plain stopped noticing it was even there, even though it was right there, right in front of me!

During my recovery, when I started sitting at my window and noticing the birds, animals, insects and even the trees, I became quite overwhelmed by how much of this amazing world I had been missing out on. It was right there in my garden and my street. I would sit for hours watching the birds and the squirrels coming and going in the garden and how the garden changed throughout the seasons. This in turn, meant that I started to notice more about what was going on inside my home as well as outside. I became so grateful for everything and everyone in my life, and although I wasn't fit enough to do the things I used to do, I was honestly so thankful for what I could do, see and notice. It's amazing what a small shift in thinking can do to our overall happiness and appreciation of life. Nothing else had changed, only my perspective, and wow, what a difference that had made!

Sometimes it can feel a bit hard to start practicing gratitude, especially when we have been unwell or struggling in some way for a time. However, once you get going things get easier, because the more you are in the attitude of gratitude, the more things you see and experience to be grateful for.

I found it was easier to start small and work my way up. This could be that you are grateful for the food you have been able to prepare and eat yourself, the water coming from the taps, the supermarket for delivering your groceries, the bin men for taking away your rubbish (and recycling it), having a shower today, a card that came in the post or cuddles with your pets (unless it's a fish – that might not be good for them!) My point is, if you break it down, you'll soon find lots of small things to be grateful for that would usually go unnoticed.

If you get into the habit of writing down at least three or maybe even five things at the end of each day that you are grateful for, then you'll soon have too many things to write down each day!

It's worth remembering, as I said before, that what we focus on flourishes. If we keep focusing on what we don't want or have, then we'll simply reinforce these very things in our life. However, if we make a conscious effort to spend at least some of our day, every day, focusing on what we do have, then those things will get reinforced instead. And, the attitude of gratitude always means you'll find more things to be grateful for!

You could write down your gratitude list in your phone or on your computer, in a notebook, or on scraps of paper and place them in a gratitude jar, and empty the jar to read these once a year. Or you could get one of the many really lovely gratitude journals out there. There are even beautiful versions of these journals for children. They can draw and write what they are grateful for, instilling happy, positive habits, memories and creating keepsakes about gratitude from a young age. And they'll have fun while doing it!

Resources

Way of the Peaceful Warrior - **Dan Millman**

A Simple Act of Gratitude - **John Kralik**

My First Gratitude Journal, A Write-in, Draw-in Gratitude Journal for Kids - **Vivian Tenorio**

Gratitude: A Daily Journal - Inspiring You To Make The Miracle Of Gratitude Part Of Your Daily Life - **Clare Josa**

Buddha Doodles Gratitude Journal: Shining Your Light - **Molly Hahn**

The Secret Gratitude Book - **Rhonda Byrne**

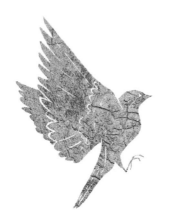

CHAPTER 4

SELF-TALK AND SELF-LOVE

How people treat you is their karma;
how you react is yours – **Wayne W Dyer**

How do you feel about yourself? How often do you mentally beat yourself up? How many times have you called yourself stupid, forgetful, fat, thin, dumb or subjected yourself to other negative thoughts like this? If you're anything like I was, then this has been the background (and sometimes the foreground) dialogue to your life.

If you're still doing this, then you may not be aware that this negative way of thinking about yourself does more than just make you more miserable and self-hating. Well, it does. It not only reinforces your negative habits, but it also becomes a self-fulfilling prophecy! Chemical, and thus physical reactions are produced in your body every time you self-talk in this way.

In Bruce Lipton's book, *The Biology of Belief,* he explains the exact science behind how this works, how it affects our cells and the way negative thoughts behave and work in our bodies. Negative thinking creates and reinforces the neurological pathways within the brain, making it easier to think in this way every time. It creates chemical reactions within the body which, believe it or not, can actually make us fat, thin, bold, grey - or just old. So what you believe really is what you become!

But wait! The good news is: this also works for positive thoughts too!

For instance, have you seen articles about elderly runners completing marathons, or stories of terminal cancer patients defying all odds? Well, these aren't just miracles, or people getting lucky; these are people who actually believe in themselves and their lives, and so their brain chemistry, their cellular community and their entire bodies follow suit. In his book, *It's the Thought that Counts,* David Hamilton explains how our body is hardwired to register every thought we think and every emotion we feel, how these emotions affect our overall health and how making small changes to the way we think about everyday occurrences can have a deep impact on illness, disease and pain. He also talks at length in his many books about the placebo effect and how we can 'trick' ourselves into being well, just from believing in a pill, potion, treatment or remedy.

Who says when you're old you have to be frail? You do!

And who says you're fat, thin, lazy or stupid? You do!

You are the master of your own destiny, and whatever you keep telling yourself day in and day out, then that's what's going to happen to you. You can't keep saying the same thing over and over again to yourself and not expect yourself to listen.

What you focus on flourishes, so what is it you are focusing on and what is it you actually want to flourish?

Here's one of the many ways I noticed how powerful self-talk is...

I always thought I was bad with names. I always said this to myself, over and over again, and even said it to others when I met them (as an excuse for when I inevitably forgot their name). But guess what? One day I decided to see what would happen if I stopped saying this to myself and actually started saying I was good at remembering names. You already know where this is going, don't you? I walked up to someone and said to myself that I'm good with names - and so I was - and not just half an hour later, but a day, and then many months later, I still remembered their name!

Admittedly, some of us need a little help along the way to feeling good about ourselves, but that help doesn't come from outside. It's not the new clothes, the new man, the new job, the new home or even the new diet. All these things can be nice, but they generally don't last, not over the long term, and they won't give you lasting happiness.

The only way to see permanent, and more importantly, authentic results is to be kind to yourself and start talking to and about yourself as you would wish others to talk to and about you. When you are kinder to yourself and stop giving yourself a hard time about everything, you start to let go of the negativity that you feel surrounds your life. You understand that you need time for yourself, that you are just as important (if not more important) than anyone else in your life, and that the toxic way you think about yourself is neither helpful, nor a productive way to focus your time and energy.

You start to be able to do things you never thought you could, you open your heart and life to new and exciting people and events, and you work in conjunction with your authentic self, becoming peaceful, centred, and aligned with your goals and path in life. This also has a knock-on effect on your health. You realise you are worth spending time on, nourishing yourself with good food, exercise, giving yourself rest periods, pampering sessions and doing all those things you have always promised you will do for yourself.

Cheryl Richardson's book, *The Art of Extreme Self-Care: Transform Your Life One Month at a Time,* is a wonderful, easy-to-read, and practical step-by-step guide to caring for yourself. It offers practical hints and tips about the way we talk to and about ourselves and the way we interact with others, and shows us how important it is to put ourselves first. After all, if we don't look after ourselves, then we'll not be able look after those we care for either.

I know this all may seem a little tricky, but it really is simply about forming new habits. So, let's start with the basics and work from there.

If I asked you to list all the things you didn't like about yourself, then I'm sure that you would have a pre-prepared list of these running on a loop in your mind. But what if I were to ask you what you liked about yourself? What then? Can you think of anything? If you have deep negativity about yourself, you might be finding this a little hard, upsetting, or even find yourself saying things like, 'There's nothing I like about myself'.

Well, I'm here to tell you that that's just not true.

Let's try this little experiment:

Do you like your toes? If not, how about your ankles, elbows, eyes, eyebrows, lips, ears, hair, hands, arms, or your bum? I bet you like at least one of them, don't you? How about your ability to listen to others? Care for others? The love you have for your family? Do you have a natural ability with numbers? Do you have a good eye for detail? Are you passionate? A good cook? Do you work hard? You may not like the way you feel people use you, but doesn't that mean you're a good, caring and loving person if you allow this to happen?

Do you see what I'm getting at? One trick is to start making mental and/or physical lists about the things you're good, or even great at, and focus on these instead of what you perceive to be your negative traits.

Once you have started with the small things, start making the list longer and bolder. Then pick bigger and more important things about yourself. Underline what you're really good at or that you really like about yourself, highlighting or colouring them in.

Once you've done this, give these things more importance in your mind by renaming them with bolder titles. So, if you like your lips, call them your luscious lips. If you are good at quizzes then call yourself a quiz kid. If you are a good cook then call yourself a master chef. You may feel a little silly at this point but keep going. I bet you can't help but smile at some of the things you write down: they will make you happy and will help you to honestly see that you have many powerful and positive things about yourself that you do actually like.

Keep this list with you at all times. Add to the list, as and when you think of something else. Open it up and read it when you're feeling low and negative about yourself and give yourself a laugh.

I think learning to love myself was one of the hardest things I have ever done! I actually never thought it was possible for me (a bad belief there). But I did, and I do, and it's been one of the greatest gifts I could have ever given myself.

When I realised my unhappy thoughts were reinforcing the very things I disliked about my body and life, that helped a little, because it made me at least stop being quite so negative about myself, but it didn't help me actually *love* myself. That part was harder! That part took acceptance, forgiveness, courage, many reminders and gentleness.

Living in a constant state of conflict with my body and my life was exhausting, it was depleting on every level and I missed out on so many things as I wanted to hide away, or at least not be on show.

But, as I started to concentrate on the small things about myself I could agree were ok, these things grew a little, and as I started to follow my passions in life, I found I was stronger in the areas that mattered to me. For instance, I'm a great hill walker, but running, gyming (yep, this is so a word now) and cycling weren't my strong points. But now I didn't need them to be as I had other strengths that I really enjoyed. The same with yoga: I'm great at it as long as I listen to my body, don't push myself and remember to breathe. If I push myself, or try hard to achieve and look like others and give myself a hard time, then it's no good for me; I hurt myself and I don't enjoy it.

Another example of this struggle was my desire to be a writer. I knew that, due to my dyslexia, I write in a very simple and often muddled way, not in a beautiful, poetic, inspiring way as I thought other people wrote. So, for a long while I just believed I would never be a writer. But, I was so passionate about sharing with others the knowledge I'd gathered so they may not have to struggle as much as I had, that I just started to write anyway. And, what happened was that some of my readers started saying to me they loved my stuff, because it was simple and to the point - YAY!

What I am trying to get at is that if you listen to yourself, really listen and just be you, just follow what fills you up, what makes you *you*, then you quickly find that when you let go of the mask you've been hiding behind, you are happier with your life and have more energy for the things you are passionate about. When we stop trying to fit in and instead start being real, then we attract more people like us to ourselves. But when we are wearing a mask, we attract others who are wearing masks, and then relationships in our lives get complicated and we wonder why.

In my book *Loving Yourself Inside and Out,* I go into detail about many ways you can learn to love yourself and your life, and stop fighting who and what you are. But, my main share with you to start this process is this: listen to your heart. If you love to play the flute, but a parent or teacher said you were rubbish, then do it anyway. If you love to paint but don't bother because you think it's a waste of time and won't make you money, do it anyway. If you love to walk but think you should be 'gyming', walk anyway. If you enjoy cooking but think it's a waste as it's only you, then do it anyway.

Following what lights us up, what's true to who we are, is so very important to our mental, and thus our physical health. It moves us away from the people-pleasing, overachieving or trying-to-fit-in-ing (yep, I made up another word) and instead towards nourishing and nurturing pastimes for ourselves that make us feel full, and replenish us too.

Don't let anyone else's opinions put you off being who you want to be and listening to what your heart desires. I remember when I stopped partying, I thought I would turn boring and wouldn't have any friends any more. However, what happened was I had more time, energy and money to go on mini and major adventures. Walking trips, world travel and alternative events gave me the chance to meet my real self, as well as other like-minded lovelies who I could be even more of myself with.

If your heart yearns to do something else, to make a change, then follow it, because there you will be able to explore what makes you *you*, and you will also find your flock.

If you can start to accept who you are, who you are yearning to be, then the parts of yourself you struggle with won't seem so important because there's a passion in your life for other things, and you'll find your strength, courage and energy there, which in turn means things will change.

It's a little crazy that acceptance of what *is*, is the only time that things really change, because we release all those resources that have been tied up in fighting ourselves and our lives so they can work with the things that really matter to us instead.

The reason I included the topic of self-love in this book about living a less toxic life is because I have found that this lack of self-love is behind many mental and physical health concerns. But, once we address it, it's soooo much easier to make long-term and sustainable health and wellness choices for ourselves instead. When we are doing all the 'body work' which a lot of this book is made up of, but don't work with the mind and heart, then we generally only get so far with things, because when we live in a state of conflict in our minds, it doesn't create a healing place within our bodies.

Resources

The Art of Extreme Self-Care : Transform Your Life One Month at a Time - **Cheryl Richardson**

The Biology of Belief - **Bruce Lipton**

It's The Thought That Counts - **David Hamilton**

How Your Mind Can Heal Your Body - **David Hamilton**

Loving Yourself Inside & Out - **Faith Canter**

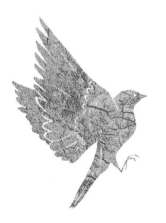

CHAPTER 5

LESS TOXIC THOUGHTS

*Don't believe everything you think – **Unknown***

It's one thing to reduce the amount of toxic thoughts and feelings we have each day, but what about the deep-seated thoughts and emotions, and the mental merry-go-rounds we sit ourselves on? How do we deal with them and how do we get off the merry-go-round?

There are many different ways we could approach deeply engrained and traumatic toxic thoughts, feelings and emotions. It really depends on who you talk to or what book you pick up - everyone has their own ideas about it. One thing everyone does seem to agree on though, is that those things won't just simply go away by themselves - you do have to do something to release them to get out of the toxic thought cycle.

When you feel constantly stressed and anxious, it impacts on your whole endocrine system (your hormones, mood, energy levels, weight and overall health). Dr James Wilson explains the exact science behind this in his book, *Adrenal Fatigue: The 21st Century Stress Syndrome.* Briefly, when we are stressed or anxious, we go into the 'fight or flight' response (as mentioned in the previous chapters), and this then causes the body to produce too much adrenaline and cortisol. This in turn interferes with the other hormones in the body, affecting insulin levels and thyroid function. It also means that the body has a harder time trying to deal with, store and/or eliminate the additional hormones released by this response.

So, my hormones were all over the show: my thyroid started to play up and, unknown to me, my adrenal glands were running in the fight or flight response over and over again, putting them under a huge amount of stress. I went down the path of trying to do something to break this internal loop of anxiety-ridden, toxic thoughts.

Emotional Freedom Technique (EFT) / Tapping

One of the most successful things I tried very early on, and which I still use regularly to this day, is Emotional Freedom Techniques (EFT). It is also called Tapping. If you have never heard of this, here is a brief overview.

EFT was founded by Gary Craig and makes use of acupuncture points (but without the needles!) With the tips of your fingers, you tap on certain points on the body whilst verbalising areas of concern; this releases the blockages created in the body by toxic thoughts. The hold these thoughts have over us is then released and most importantly, patterns associated with these thoughts are broken. It's like a counselling session but without having to open up to someone about your darkest and deepest thoughts.

For it to work most effectively, you take yourself back to the first time you had the issue or concern and tap about how this made you feel, both physically and emotionally. If you can address the root cause of the concern, then all the other times this has affected you since then will most likely be addressed in this session also. It is an extremely powerful tool and can release a lot of hurt, negative emotions, toxic thoughts and long-standing negative beliefs about yourself and others. This not only has positive psychological benefits, but it helps all sorts of physical issues that were created and/or exacerbated by these underlying thought patterns. It can help anything from back pain and weight loss to your love life and depression.

If you look up EFT / Tapping, you might get confused by all the different types and methods you find. Please don't be put off; you can keep it simple, in fact that's how I teach and use it now and it's super-effective this way as we actually tap on the thoughts and feelings, not what we *think* we should be tapping on instead.

The traditional way of tapping

1. Think about something that is bothering you, but be specific. 'I am stressed' would not be detailed enough: you need to list the reasons why and how this is affecting your body and mind. Does it make you feel sick in the tummy, tight in your chest, tearful, drained, scared, and so on?

2. For the sake of this exercise, let's name your issue 'tension in my neck'. Rate the level of intensity of the tension in your neck on a scale of 0-10 (10 being the worst).

3. Next we put together a set-up phrase. The set-up phrase focuses the mind on your issue.

4. Repeat your chosen set-up phrase three times: *'Even though I'm feeling tension in my neck, I deeply and completely love and accept myself.'*

5. Tap on lots of tapping points (on meridians of the body) while repeating reminder phrases. Reminder phrases are all the ways the tension in your neck has made you feel, both physically and emotionally.

6. If other things pop into your mind whilst you are tapping whether related or unrelated, tap on those also. More often than not, you'll be surprised to find that what pops up is very related.

7. If you can remember the first time you felt this sort of stress, then it's important to tap on that time and all the thoughts and feelings around that time. This will help all the other times since, including the one you're going through now.

8. After a couple of rounds of tapping, pause, take three deep belly breaths and notice the effects. Then reassess the intensity level. Has the number changed? What is it now? If it has dropped then you're on the right track. If it hasn't, then there's something else you should be tapping on. What could that be? What's REALLY upsetting you?

9. If the rating you now give it has dropped, but is not down to zero, refocus on your issue and repeat the tapping process again. The second time around, you can change the wording of your set-up phrase to

something like: '*Even though I still have some of this tension in my neck, I deeply and completely love and accept myself.*'

10. Then say things like: '*This remaining tension in my neck makes me feel/hurts/is* etc...' (adding any new feelings, both mental and physical about this issue).

11. After several more rounds of tapping, you should find the intensity of the feelings reduced to zero. If you stop making progress, then sit and think about what else could be affecting this issue (however small or irrelevant) and tap on that as well.

12. Either way, it is important to try to finish your tapping on a positive rather than a negative. So, consider saying things like:

- ❋ Even though I haven't got to the bottom of this issue I am open to addressing it and know I will find a way to help myself.

- ❋ I am open to healing both mentally and physically.

- ❋ I now let go of my attachments to these issues.

- ❋ These feelings do not serve me; I let go of them now.

- ❋ I thank my body and/or mind for protecting me, but they can let go of this pain now.

- ❋ Even though I find this issue too upsetting to deal with now, I know I am on the right track and I allow myself to be open and willing to heal.

The above way of tapping is effective and is also how I started to aid my own healing. However, I have also found it can be a little over-complicated at times and it can get a bit heady and robotic too.

What I have since found to be super-effective is what I call 'the easy way to tap'. This way, we generally just focus on the one tapping point (or more if that resonates with you too). I like to use the 'Karate Chop' point (see image on following pages). This one can be used anywhere, even if you are sat in traffic which is when many people start to get stressed and agitated.

This easy way of tapping is about working on raw emotions *in the moment*. When we work with our thoughts, feelings and emotions like this, we can have big shifts, quickly, because we are 'in it'; it's raw, it's true and it's not thinking about what we think we need to tap on, but instead what is already going on for us in our heads. This way, we just tap on our exact thoughts, unedited, swear words 'n all.

I know this can sound kind of backwards to a lot of alternative practices and ideas, because instead of trying to think, say or do something in a positive way, (like positive affirmations), we are doing the opposite. We are voicing or honouring our perceived negative thoughts. For me, this is super-important and powerful. Having spent a lifetime trying to be positive and not understanding why I never succeeded for very long, I can see why. Because I was pushing parts of me away, not honouring the bits than made me *me*. If you are saying a million positive things to yourself every day, but on the inside doing the opposite, then you are going to cause yourself a whole load of conflict, stress and anxiety instead.

So, we tap on all the crappy thoughts and feelings and then when we have got those out, we put in some good stuff. But again, we don't go from saying things like 'I hate my body and life' to 'I love my body and life', because of course, this will cause conflict, unless we really believe it. The better approach here is to use words like 'permission' or 'open'. What I mean by this is, instead of saying, 'I love my body and life' (unless you believe it), I would recommend saying, 'I am open to loving my body and life' or 'I give myself permission to love my body and life'. This sends a powerful message to the subconscious mind that maybe you are open to doing just that.

Giving ourselves permission is an important one, especially if we have been ill for a long time. When I was chronically ill with ME/CFS, giving myself permission to be well again seemed to create a big shift in me. I was so used to being ill and its label, that giving myself permission to be something else was big.

The positive tapping at the end of the process should incorporate some of the negative stuff you said at the beginning. So, if you said things like *'I am broken / incomplete / need fixing / fat / thin / screwed up'*, then the positive bits at the end could be something like:

I am open to not feeling broken any more / I give myself permission to feel complete / I am open to not feeling like I need fixing / I give myself permission to love my body / I am open to not feeling screwed up, or even, I give myself permission to be ok with feeling screwed up.

You can also add in things that resonate all of a sudden that have nothing to do with what you are tapping on.

So, to recap:

- ❀ Pick a tapping point or points that feel right for you. You can look up the traditional points online.

- ❀ You tap on your raw emotions, feelings or thoughts in the moment (even if that means running off to the toilet for a 30 second tap because a work colleague has upset you).

- ❀ And, when I say raw emotions, feelings or thoughts, I even mean ones like: 'Faith doesn't know what she is talking about, tapping sucks and makes me feel silly and I really don't get how it's meant to help.' Or even: 'I have no idea what to tap on, I'm just feeling crappy' (then follow with why you feel crappy and tap on this). You tap on any resistances to tapping too!

- ❀ Tap until you have got it all out.

- ❀ Tap on being open or giving yourself permission to letting go, moving through or thinking another way about your situation and do that until it feels right and finished too.

- ❀ Then, just like the traditional way of tapping, take some deep breaths to let go and ground yourself with.

I have noticed that sometimes when you finish, you may feel there's something else you want to tap on and of course, you can start again with that. But, one of the main things you may find at this point is that you are crying, coughing, yawning, feeling edgy or jittery, or feeling energised or tired. These are all fine, and generally it means the body and mind are letting go. If you don't feel anything though, that's totally ok too; sometimes it takes a while for the energy to start moving.

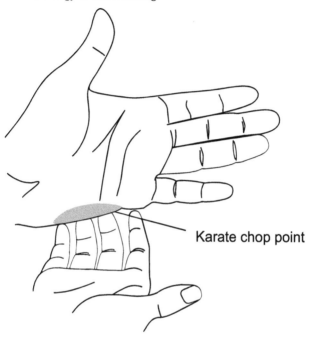

Karate chop point

Forgiveness

*When you forgive, you in no way change the past, but you sure do change the future – **Bernard Meltzer***

Most people agree that forgiveness is part of the healing process: this could be forgiving yourself or someone else. Learning to forgive can be tricky, and although many people have tried to practise forgiveness and many books have been written about it, sometimes this can take time and perseverance. Sometimes, it's just the right approach at just the right time. Either way, I believe that there is a way forward for all of us.

Personally, I used to find it hard to forgive. I couldn't forgive myself. I realise now that some bad things had to happen for me to become the person that I am, but I simply could not forgive the people who had made them happen. I didn't see why I had to. I felt justified in my thoughts, feelings and anger. Everyone talked about forgiveness and how it helped you heal, but I thought, 'Well, they clearly haven't been through what I've been through then, have they?'

I eventually realised that that this cycle of anxiety, stress and toxic thoughts wasn't doing me any good: in fact it was helping to keep me incredibly ill. But I still felt justified in my feelings; they were my feelings and I was wronged, so I could feel this way, right?

I struggled with the concept of forgiveness for many years. How could a person possibly forgive someone who had destroyed their life? How could they forgive themselves if they had wronged someone else?

I read many books, talked to many people and researched this concept as much as possible, but nothing ever quite sank in: I just didn't get it! I did know that this cycle of toxic thoughts wasn't affecting anyone else but myself, that I was still in 'victim mode', still allowing the people that had hurt me to have some sort of control over my life, and that this wasn't acceptable either.

Then I realised that it wasn't the bad things other people did to me, or the bad I things that I did to them that was the issue. It was the lack of respect I had for myself that was the issue. Without respect, there is no love; without love, there is no forgiveness, and without forgiveness there is no escape from toxic thoughts.

So here's what I did.

I seemed to know intuitively I had to find a quiet spot. I closed my eyes and asked myself what I could really do for myself, what I wanted and how I could help myself heal. The response I got quite clearly was, 'Let go, move on and open your heart to love for yourself, just as you open it to others.'

I used EFT / tapping to do this. I tapped on forgiving myself, reasons why I didn't respect and like myself, and forgiving that small child within me for not knowing any better. I also tapped on allowing myself to be open to forgiveness, that 'Even though I may not be able to do this right now, I am open to this idea and I am open to respecting and loving myself more.' I also used visual-isations and meditations of filling my whole body with healing, loving, forgiving light. I started to talk to and about myself (and also about others) in a much more positive and kinder way and I allowed myself to be open to the universe, (God, source, love or whatever you like to call it.) I basically taught myself to let go, to let go of the hurt, the anger, the pain and the finger-pointing.

I then had an epiphany and realised that every awful thing I'd been through in my life was for a purpose. At the time these events had happened, they hurt so much that I wasn't in a position to see them for what they were. I had always felt sorry for myself and the things I had gone through in my short life, but today I can honestly say that I no longer do. I have learnt from all the people who treated me badly, from my illnesses and from my past. I now know this was part of my own path, and that path has led me to be where I am now.

As for forgiving, once I learnt to love and respect myself, it was much easier to forgive myself, and of course, once I could forgive myself, it was easier to forgive others. None of us are perfect, we all make mistakes, and for the most part, this is how we learn. Sometimes it's good to feel bad if we've upset someone, but getting stuck in the space of guilt, denial or hate is not healthy for anyone. And it only really harms you and not the person who you feel has done you wrong. Once you start to respect yourself, you understand that it's only really *you* who's punishing you. You see that you can let go of these thoughts and feelings. And when you open yourself up to love, there is less and less room for those pesky toxic thoughts.

Why not try some EFT or tapping today on being open to forgiving, to moving on, to loving and respecting yourself and others? Even if you don't feel quite ready to actually forgive right now, or to move on, or to let go, or to love and respect yourself more, then you can still tap on being open to this prospect happening in the future. This might be all you need to open the door to this new journey of letting go.

Resources

Loveability - **Robert Holden**

Billy - **Pamela Stevenson**

The Journey: An Extraordinary Guide to Healing Your Life and Setting Yourself Free - **Brandon Bays**

The EFT Manual - **Gary Craig**

The Tapping Solution - **Nick Ortner**

The Breakthrough Experience - **Dr John F. Demartini**

www.bachcentre.com

www.faithcanter.com/videos

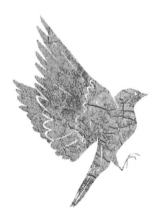

CHAPTER 6

LESS TOXIC BODIES

Eliminate what does not help you evolve – **Unknown**

Most of us are pretty toxic beings, we have maybe spent a lifetime putting things into our bodies that we assumed were ok for us because they are sold in most of the shops we visit. However, this couldn't be further from the truth. The fact is, many of the items we purchase, from food and drink to toiletries and cleaning products, are highly toxic to us (and of course the environment). It benefits pretty much all mental and physical health concerns if we work towards expelling these toxins from our lives.

It's important to remember that when detoxing your body and mind, the correct support is essential throughout the process. This ensures effective detoxification, as well as minimising side effects.

There is something to remember when considering a quick-fix detox: your body couldn't deal with, or eliminate, the high level of toxins the first time it took them on board, which is why they have been stored in your body. So, be careful with the kind of detox you pick to address your toxic load.

If you feel you may have a high level of toxins in your body and you decide to only do a quick-fix detox, it is likely you'll go through terrible detox symptoms, only to absorb most of these toxins right back into your body again. As you can imagine, this is pretty pointless: it's a massive strain on the body, and to top it all off, you make yourself feel worse without any real long-term benefits.

In my personal experience, and those of my clients, I have found that slow and steady always wins the race when it comes to detoxing and general good health. The more you support your body when detoxing, and in particular the liver and lymphatic system, the more effective and less traumatic it will be.

It's also true that, if you have a terrible diet, use lots of toxins in your home and on your body, and are generally overloaded by toxic thoughts and feelings, you cannot 'fix' this by detoxing for one or two weeks out of the year. It might help you lose weight or give you a bit more energy for a short time, but for the most part, all you are doing is shifting toxins around. A better course of action is to look at your daily routine and slowly remove or exchange one toxic item for a less toxic one.

However, when toxins leave your system, even with a slow and gentle approach, the process can still make you feel a little under the weather. It is perfectly normal to feel a little rotten, sweat a little more, feel tired, achy, headachy and go to the toilet more often. This is actually a good thing as your body is trying to expel the toxins through the proper channels.

The more you can do during this particular time, (and subsequently, of course), to reduce the amount of toxins absorbed by your body, the better you will feel.

The key points for expelling toxins permanently from the body are:

1. Reduce the toxic load in your food. Replace processed sugars and white foods (like bread, flour and rice) with wholemeal versions and stay clear of sweeteners, diet foods and drinks, and caffeine and alcohol.

2. Reduce the use of chemical toxins in your home and on your body. Your body absorbs a lot of the toxins from its environment, so replace these with natural alternatives or make your own (see later chapters).

3. Drink plenty of water, at least 2-3 litres every day (and more, if exercising). Make sure you drink from a non-plastic, or at least a BPA-free plastic container. This will help your lymphatic system eliminate toxins.

4. Ideally, drink at least a litre of water as soon as you wake up, and before doing anything else with your day.

5. Exercise regularly. This doesn't need to be high impact – just a minimum of 20 minutes, four times a week. This helps your body sweat out toxins.

6. Increase your intake of probiotic foods and drinks. Here, I mean fermented (not pickled) vegetables and drinks such as kefir and kombucha: these are an amazing source of many billions of different probiotic bacteria. These bacteria help the body eliminate toxins, and balance good and bad bacteria and yeasts in the gut. Failing this, take a really good quality, multi-strain

probiotic supplement (one which contains many billions of multi-strain good bacteria).

7. Support your body, and in particular the liver, with appropriate herbs and natural remedies. Burdock, parsley, peppermint, turmeric, black walnut, elderberry, dandelion, nettle, liverwort, wormwood, charcoal and milk thistle all help the body to detox and support the liver through the detoxification process. The more bitter, the better!

8. Increase your consumption of magnesium-rich foods (leafy greens, nuts, seeds, beans, lentils, fish, avocados, figs, bananas and whole grains). Try to also have as many Epsom salt baths as possible. Epsom salts are high in magnesium and help to draw out toxins. They also help with general aches and pains, so they are great after exercising. You should be in the bath for a minimum of 20 minutes (relaxing!) for an optimum effect.

9. Consider regular massage, reflexology, Rolfing, saunas, steam rooms or any other detoxifying therapies. These therapies stimulate the lymphatics, helping them to eliminate toxins through our skin and via our urine.

10. Take up body brushing. You can use a long-handled brush or just your own hands and brush your body in the direction of the chest. And ladies: please make sure that you brush *up* the sides of your breasts, towards the area just above the breast, as a lot of toxins are

stored in breast tissue. They may become tender once you start shifting toxins, but keep going as that's a good sign and the tenderness will disappear. Body-brushing stimulates the lymphatics and removes blockages.

11. Don't skip meals. Eating regularly means your body can work more effectively, and when this happens, you eliminate toxins better. An additional benefit: your blood sugar levels won't get so low that you feel the need to snack on something naughty!

12. Make sure you are having at least one bowel movement each day. Bowel movements are one of the body's main ways to remove toxins. If you're not having at least one bowel movement a day, then a lot of toxins are being held in your body. This will mean that you will be re-absorbing these toxins. If you're not having regular bowel movements, try eating more fibre, drinking more water, and take up body-brushing and rebounding (jumping on a mini trampoline).

13. Try daily rebounding as this helps stimulate the lymphatics.

14. Try not to use antiperspirants. These products impair the body's ability to eliminate toxins through sweating. I know some people worry about body odour, so they still use antiperspirant products. If nothing else, try to cut them out when you are at home to allow your body to sweat normally. If the toxins can't get out, they will be stored in your body. There are a lot of great natural

products on the market (my favourite is PitRock, a salt stone deodorant). Once your body has eliminated the build-up of toxins and you have lowered your toxic intake, you won't need a deodorant because you won't smell when you sweat. Bad body odour is caused by toxins leaving the body. That's why people smell worse after a drinking session, a takeaway or when on medication.

15. Try to get a minimum of eight hours' sleep a night. Your body does a lot of its detoxing during the night, so it's important to give it enough time and energy to do this.

16. When eating meat and dairy, always try to opt for organic versions so you will be absorbing fewer toxins.

17. If you don't understand the ingredients list in a food, avoid it. Strange words on labels usually mean chemicals, and they will only add to your toxic load.

18. Look into the symptoms of a yeast imbalance in the gut. When bad yeasts grow, they create an imbalance in the body. This produces toxins that the body eliminates. This can make us feel pretty lousy. However, it's fairly simple to bring the good and bad yeasts back into balance by changing your diet, adding some natural antifungal foods to your meals, and increasing your consumption of fermented/probiotic foods and drinks (more details about this later in the book).

19. Breathe deeply and fully into the lungs, stomach and back, with purpose, as many times in the day as

possible. As previously mentioned, this will help your body remove toxins from the respiratory system and allow the rest of your body to get the energy and oxygen it requires to do its job effectively.

20. Try to incorporate yoga, pilates, t'ai chi, qigong or meditation into your daily life. These activities will help support and strengthen your body and mind for detoxification and much more.

21. Swap your normal fluoride toothpastes and mouthwashes for more natural non-fluoride versions. Consider having mercury fillings removed by someone who specialises in this process.

22. Consume detoxing clays like bentonite or liquid zeolites. These bind to toxins and ensure they are expelled from the body rather than reabsorbed.

23. And finally, reduce your stress levels! High stress levels lead to an overproduction of hormones such as cortisol and adrenaline. When this happens, many of the normal functions of the body are impaired and this can mean that, not only are you not eliminating toxins, but you're also storing these additional hormones. When you're stressed, you tend not to eat well, exercise or generally look after yourself as you should.

Resources

Qi Gong for Beginners - **Stanley D. Wilson**

Teach Yourself Meditation - **Eric Harrison**

Fast Food Nation - **Eric Schlosser**

Not on the Label - **Felicity Lawrence**

The Gerson Therapy: The Proven Nutritional Program for Cancer and Other Illnesses – **Charlotte Gerson and Morton Walker**

The pH Miracle: Balance Your Diet, Reclaim Your Health - **Robert O. Young & Shelley Redford Young**

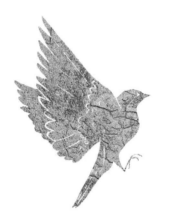

CHAPTER 7

FOODIE FACTS

*One cannot think well, love well and sleep well if one
has not dined well – **Virginia Woolf***

I'm pretty sure we've all got a good idea of what we should and shouldn't be doing when it comes to food. So why don't we do it?

Some of the reasons are: convenience, addiction, food producers' marketing strategies, and thinking healthy food doesn't taste good and costs a lot. There are also emotionally-related food habits (which can be dealt with by following some of the steps in the previous chapters of this book).

We all live busy, usually stress-filled lives and we don't really appreciate how what we are putting into our bodies has an effect on, not just the health of our bodies, but the health of our minds too. If we could see the effects of the harmful foods and drinks on our insides, we would think again. Processed and chemically-laden foods cause diabetes, cancers, auto-immune diseases, food sensitivities, IBS, depression, anxiety, not to mention weight gain and poor absorption of vitamins and minerals (leading to a whole host of other issues). Most of us know this, but most of us still eat these foods.

It doesn't help that a lot of processed foods appear to be cheaper than healthy food. When watching our spending, we are often are drawn to processed foods because of this. However, if you batch-cook your meals (i.e., make up enough for say ten meals in one go), you not only save yourself time over the coming weeks by not cooking individual meals, but you also save yourself money, as this does work out a lot cheaper than buying individual pre-packed, processed meals.

Everyone knows that alcohol, cigarettes and caffeine are addictive, but most people give little thought to the fact that sugars, sweeteners, carbohydrates, glutens and salts can be just as addictive. We either buy foods which already contain the latter, or we add them to our foods further down the line in the form of sauces, dips, dressings and condiments.

Sugars, carbohydrates, glutens and anything high on the Glycaemic Index (GI) produce chemical reactions within the body and brain when we eat them. These chemical reactions make us feel happy and satisfied and those feelings are what the body becomes addicted to: so much so that we actually crave them. What's more, the more of these foods we eat, the more our hormones become imbalanced (especially our insulin levels) and the more our bodies crave them. It's a vicious circle and the only real way to deal with this is to exchange bad for good and break the habits and the cravings.

*

FOOD	RECOMMENDATION
White rice	Brown rice or quinoa
White processed sugars and sweeteners	Honey (preferably raw) or Maple syrup
White flours	Wholemeal flours (or gluten-free flours)
Bread	Sourdough bread
White potatoes	Sweet potatoes
Margarine	Organic butter (yes, a little butter is actually better for you than trans-fat margarines)
Sunflower and vegetable oils (more nasty trans-fats)	Coconut oil (or olive oil for dressings and low temperature cooking)
Monosodium glutamate (MSG)	Just about any other herb, spice or flavouring
Caffeine-based drinks	Rooibos tea (caffeine-free) or even green tea (which still has caffeine in it, but it also has a lot of positive health benefits)
Fizzy drinks	Kombucha (it's just like a soda) or even sparkling water with a squeeze of fresh fruit
Store-bought juices, smoothies and concentrates	Homemade juice direct from the fruit, without the added sugars, sweeteners and preservatives (it has a much higher nutritional content)
High-sugar fruits (dried fruits, bananas, grapes, pineapples, etc.)	If you eat masses of high sugar fruits, they will make your blood sugars fluctuate a lot. Keep your consumption to a minimum until you have eliminated your sugar and carbohydrate cravings.
Table salt	Sea salt or Himalayan salt
Sweeteners	Honey or fresh fruit
Concentrated juice or squash	Slices of lemon, orange, lime, ginger or cucumber in water
Meat, fish and dairy	Always buy organic if you can
Vegetarian meat substitutes (like quorn, microprotein or soy)	Fermented options like bean curd or tempeh
Cooked	Raw food! Swap one cooked meal a day for one raw meal or try to have 50% of each meal raw
Ready meals	Batch cook your own and freeze it
Microwave	Standard oven or dehydrator
Boiled	Steamed

*A note on grains, lentils and pulses

Grains, lentils, beans, seeds and nuts all get a hard time. People are rightly concerned about enzyme inhibitors in nuts and seeds and nutrient inhibitors in grains, lentils and pulses. There is a simple way around releasing these inhibitors (which prevent you from absorbing all the enzymes and vitamins and minerals from these foods). This is to soak and sprout these foods before using them.

If you soak nuts and seeds and then dry them out again, not only are the enzyme inhibitors released, but the nuts and seeds themselves are much more easily digestible.

When you soak grains, lentils and pulses (changing the water regularly), until they start to sprout little tails, then you not only release the nutrient inhibitors but you also increase the nutritional content of these foods. These can then be used in the normal way (i.e., cooking with them) or you can eat them raw in salads and such, for optimum enzyme and nutrient levels.

Below is a soaking and sprouting guide for you. Please note that some items, due to the way they are harvested, are not raw, and so will not sprout.

FOOD	SOAKING TIME	SPROUTING TIME
Almonds	10 to 12 hours	3 days (only if raw)
Adzuki Beans	10 to 12 hours	4 days
Amaranth	8 to 12 hours	1 day
Black Beans	8 hours	3 days
Brazil Nuts	3 hours	will not sprout
Buckwheat	6 hours	2 days
Cashews	2 to 4 hours	will not sprout
Chia	1 hour	will not sprout
Chickpeas	8 hours	2 days
Flaxseeds	1 to 2 hours	will not sprout
Hazelnuts	8 to 12 hours	will not sprout
Lentils	7 to 10 hours	2 days
Millet	5 to 7 hours	12 hours
Mung Beans	8 to 12 hours	4 days
Oat groats	6 hours	2 days
Pecans	6 to 8 hours	will not sprout
Pistachios	8 to 10 hours	will not sprout
Pumpkin seeds	8 to 12 hours	3 days
Radish seeds	8 to 12 hours	3 days
Sesame seeds	8 hours	2 days
Sunflower seeds	8 to 12 hours	12-24 hours
Quinoa	8 to 12 hours	2 days
Walnuts	4 to 6 hours	will not sprout
Wild rice	24 to 48 hours	3 days

What are trans fats?

Trans fats are oils that have been hydrogenated (hydrogen has been added to them) for aid in the processes of preserving or solidifying food products. Trans fats can be found in many of our foods these days, but the main culprits are sunflower oil, vegetable oil and margarine.

The problem with these trans fats is that whilst we perceive them to be healthier than other natural oils and animal products like butter, etc., in actual fact, they are toxic to our system and our body cannot process them. When they enter the body, it treats them in the same way that it does a normal healthy fat and absorbs them into the cells. However, as they are processed fats, the cells have no natural way to deal with them; they are retained and the cells start to harden. The metabolic system cannot deal with this, and health conditions such as diabetes, obesity, immune system-related conditions and weight gain around the stomach are hugely impacted.

What's Monosodium Glutamate (MSG)?

MSG is a food flavouring: it intensifies the flavours in your food, and it is highly addictive and toxic. It's what makes you feel really full after eating but then, an hour later, you feel like you are starving! (Some people also notice a tingling of the lips when they have eaten a lot of this.) You may have felt this way after eating a Chinese take-away, as Chinese food often contains a lot of MSG. It has been linked to diabetes, skin conditions, mood swings, food intolerances, digestive issues, fatigue, obesity, depression, migraines, learning disabilities and dementia.

If you avoid processed and fast foods, then you will greatly reduce your MSG intake by default. However, MSG can be found in a lot of basic ingredients you buy, as it is known by many names and has the E number E621. It can be found in many yeast-based products, so be sure to read the labels carefully.

Sweeteners, anyone?

In my opinion, man-made sweeteners should be avoided at all costs. They are added to almost all processed foods, fizzy drinks, chewing gum, sweets, fruit cordials and diet foods. We have been told this is because they are lower in calories than sugar: which they are! However, because our bodies are unable to process these toxic chemicals (formaldehyde, for example) these are often stored as fat. They are related to obesity, health conditions, diabetes, depression, headaches, hormonal issues, balance issues, confusion and thyroid disease.

Much better options than man-made sweeteners are natural ones such as honey, maple syrup, agave nectar or just fresh fruit. However, if you are wanting to stabilise blood sugars or hormones, or you have diabetes, then keep your intake of even these to a minimum as they will still affect your body in a similar way to cane sugar or sweetener-based foods.

Soy?

Soy has got a bad rap recently and rightly so. In its raw form, i.e., the one you find in vegetarian foods, sauces and processed foods, it disrupts your hormones and should be kept to a bare minimum. However, in its fermented form, i.e., tofu and bean curd, it is thought to be very beneficial and even alkalising to the body. I would still recommend not eating high quantities of soy even in this form, as soy is finding its way into more and more of our food products: if you eat processed foods you probably already have too much soy in your diet.

Salt

Contrary to popular belief, you actually need salt in your diet. The problem is the type and amount of salt. Not only do almost all processed and fast foods have salt in them, but so do a great many other items that claim to be healthy. It's very easy for your salt intake to get out of hand these days. If you eat a fair amount of processed foods, then you are already getting enough salt in your diet and shouldn't be adding more to your food whilst cooking or at the table. However, if you start eating healthier meals, then your salt intake will come down by default. The body does need salt, especially if you are suffering from adrenal issues and/ or stress-related concerns. So in these instances, to cut out salt altogether would not be a good idea. The thing to do is to replace it with salts that are better for you.

My favourite salt is pink Himalyan rock salt: it's full of minerals, is strong and ever so slightly sweet so you don't need to use huge amounts. Celtic salt and any other sea salts work just as well.

Gluten

Gluten gives elasticity to dough and helps it rise and keep its shape.

This protein-like substance is another food item that gets bad press these days. Everyone thinks they are gluten-intolerant or have issues with it in general. Well, this is justified! It is thought that one in three of us has a gluten intolerance and some people even develop coeliac disease. Our bodies find it hard to process gluten, especially at the levels at which we consume it. It can lead to other food intolerances, leaky gut syndrome, depression, mood swings, blood sugar issues, IBS, skin conditions, weight gain, bloating, upset stomach, hormonal problems and auto-immune issues.

The problem is not only the high amount of gluten in our diets, but also that most of the gluten-free options are high in sugars, sweeteners, salts and preservatives, making them nowhere near as healthy as we'd like to think. Gluten consumption should be minimised where possible or, even better, cut out altogether to prevent an increased risk of digestive problems.

If you are like most of the population and love your bread, then a great alternative is sourdough, especially if you make it in a fermented way at home (more about this in the next chapter). There is no gluten in this dough and also no added chemicals or processed yeasts. It's much more like the bread we all ate many years ago (when no one had gluten intolerances). You can also make normal bread with a sourdough starter and, due to the fermentation process, the good yeasts will use and eat up both the gluten and bad yeasts to help the bread rise and form – good little yeasts!

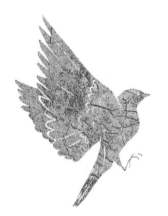

CHAPTER 8

DIGESTIVE HEALTH

*The road to health is paved with good intestines – **Sherry A. Rogers***

Traditional medicine often looks at the symptoms rather than the cause when addressing health concerns. As such, underlying health issues are often not dealt with, but instead raise their ugly heads either with the same symptoms later on down the line, or with new symptoms.

Illnesses like Crohn's disease, food intolerances, IBS, leaky gut and coeliac disease can all be repaired through good gut health. As these health concerns are all gut-based, it is not surprising that maintaining a healthy gut can aid recovery. But what if I also told you that autoimmune diseases like lupus, MS, diabetes, some forms of thyroid disease and many more autoimmune issues, skin conditions, mental health concerns, weight gain, fatigue, brain fog and some learning difficulties are also thought to be curable, or least made substantially better by addressing gut health?

When you maintain good gut health, it has a huge, positive impact on your overall health, both mentally and physically.

Here are the reasons why:

1. The toxicity of the body will be greatly reduced: the digestive system will be able to eliminate more of the

toxins from food and drink consumed and a balance of good and bad bacteria in the digestive system will be achieved. When the bad bacteria get out of hand, they create more and more toxins as they grow, raising the body's toxicity levels and putting additional strain on the lymphatics, as well as many other parts of the body. When you bring these into balance, you will find that the body eliminates these toxins easily and you feel better not only in the gut, but throughout your body.

2. With better gut health, your digestive enzyme levels are higher, enabling the body to process foods and absorb and utilise nutrients from your food.

3. Your gut is the core of the body's immune system. With better gut health, you have better health in general, and consequently, fewer illnesses.

4. We produce around 95% of our serotonin in the gut (and the rest in the brain), so good gut health means a happier you.

5. With better gut health, inflammation in the body will be greatly reduced, which helps a whole host of other health complaints, including arthritis and joint and muscular pain.

6. You'll have more energy, as the body uses up a lot of energy trying to process foods and drinks that upset the digestive system.

7. All gut-based illnesses, such as IBS, leaky gut and many more, should improve when addressing the health of the gut.

8. Brain fog, mental clarity, memory issues and mood issues can all be minimised when addressing gut health, as many of the essential enzymes, vitamins and minerals needed for these functions of the body will be absorbed and utilised more easily within the body.

As you can see, there are many benefits to good gut health, and you'll be pleased to know it's fairly easy to start achieving this. There are many pills, potions and programmes that claim to do this, but in my opinion, getting back to basics is the easiest and most effective way to do this. This means following the suggestions in the previous chapter, and introducing more raw, enzyme-rich, fermented/cultured, and probiotic-rich foods and drinks. Then lastly, allowing the digestive system (and thus the rest of the body) to detox, because if the body is full of toxins, it's not able to take on board the nutrients it requires for good health.

Raw Food

Raw food - uncooked, unprocessed, unpasteurised, mostly organic, enzyme and nutrient-rich foods.

What's are the benefits of eating more raw food?

1. You will be minimising the amount of toxins coming into your body through what you are eating and drinking.

2. When you cook food, you destroy much of its nutritional content and enzyme levels, so eating it raw, or ever so lightly warmed through, means you are more likely to benefit from all that lovely goodness which is naturally in your food.

3. Because of the increase in essential nutrients and enzymes in your food, you will find you have more energy, sleep better and think and feel better.

4. You skin, hair and nails will be healthier because more nutrients are being absorbed into your system.

5. You can pretty much eat as much as you want, as it's all healthy, hearty food.

6. You'll find yourself feeling full quicker and staying full longer as the body receives its required nutrients more quickly and is not searching or craving for more.

7. Eating fresh, nutrient-rich, energy-full foods helps ground you and gives you a better connection to the Earth.

8. And lastly, raw food tastes so delicious!

For those of you who are new to raw food, I don't just mean salads, juices and smoothies. Although these are wonderful and do count towards your raw food intake, (so you are probably already consuming more raw food than you realise), I mean so much more than this. If you are lucky enough to have a raw food supplier near you, or have purchased a dehydrator, you will find that you can make the raw equivalent of just about any cooked meal. You can do pizzas, pasta dishes, lasagnes, quiches and so much more. These dishes are made with raw, organic, fresh vegetables, nuts, seeds and fruits, and then dehydrated for many hours at a very low heat. This lightly warms the food through to create a slightly cooked effect, but the heat is not high enough to destroy the enzymes or nutrients.

You don't have to eat a fully raw diet to benefit from it. I suggest to clients that they replace one cooked meal a day with a raw one, or having half of the food on your plate raw will certainly start the ball rolling towards many of the amazing health benefits.

Many of the ingredients in the following recipes for raw meals are the same or similar or can be substituted for other things. So, although it may look like you have to buy a lot of new ingredients, once you have the basics in your store cupboard, you'll be able to make many healthy raw recipes. I recommend buying one or two new items for your larder (like some seeds, nuts or dried fruits) each time you do your shopping and before long, you'll be set to rustle up a raw food feast regularly.

In the next section, I am going to share with you many of my favourite raw food recipes. I recommend the use of a food processor or blender for many of these.

FAVOURITE RAW FOOD RECIPES

Raw Un-fried Rice

Ingredients

190g wild rice

½ head of green or red cabbage

1 red onion

1 tsp. garlic granules or 2 cloves garlic

3 tbsp. grated ginger (or half as much ground ginger)

2 heads of broccoli cut into small florets, stems peeled and shredded

2 large carrots shredded

1 sweet pepper (any colour)

1 bunch parsley chopped or 1 tbsp. of dried parsley

190g peas and/or sweetcorn (frozen and thawed)

95g lime or lemon juice

170g olive oil or your choice of oil

170g sesame oil (optional, add half as much if you are also using sesame seed oil)

½ tsp of dried flaked seaweed

1½ tsp. Himalayan salt

½ tsp. chilli pepper

Directions

1. Soak wild rice for 48 hours in water (changing water and rinsing rice every 6-8 hours).

2. If you cannot tolerate wild rice or if you want a quick and non-raw substitute, then you could use brown rice, lentils or quinoa.

3. Put all vegetables (except broccoli, peas and sweetcorn) and dressing items into a food processor and blitz until all items are the size of large peas.

4. Put mixture into a bowl, add the items you have left out, mix well and put into the fridge for 2 hours (or even better, overnight).

5. Mix well before serving.

6. If you don't have any of the above vegetables, use what you do have. This is a great 'use-up' recipe, so just about any vegetable works.

Marinated Vegetables

Ingredients

1 large courgette

1 red pepper

1 yellow pepper

1 small red onion

5 or 6 mushrooms

2 tbsp. olive oil

2 tbsp. sesame seed oil

1 tsp. flax seed oil (optional)

½ tsp. garlic granules (optional)

½ tbsp. mixed dried herbs or 50g fresh herbs chopped

Directions

1. Cut up all the vegetables or use a spiralizer (to make 'raw spaghetti' from vegetables), a mandolin or slice thinly with a knife.

2. Place these and the other ingredients in a bowl and mix well.

3. Cover and place in the fridge to marinate for at least 2 hours, but preferably overnight.

Pizza

Ingredients for the base

90g ground buckwheat

570g chopped celery

120g ground flaxseed

2 tbsp. olive oil

½ tsp. Himalayan rock salt

200-250ml water

Directions

1. Add all the ingredients to a food processor and blend until the mixture resembles a batter.

2. Form one or two large pizza bases or several smaller ones (you will get about 14 from this recipe) on a waxed dehydrator sheet. Simply dollop some mix on the sheet and using the back of a spoon, spread it out evenly in circles (the bases will shrink slightly on cooking, so it's better to make them slightly bigger than you require). If you are having difficulty spreading the mix, then return it to the blender and add a little more water.

3. Place on a tray in a dehydrator (which warms food through without destroying enzymes or nutrients) at 104°F/40°C for 5-6 hours and then turn them over, placing them directly on the tray without the waxed dehydrator sheet.

4. Dehydrate for another 6-8 hours until fairly firm.

Toppings

1. Either use the tomato pasta sauce recipe in this book, or roughly blend a few tomatoes with some mixed herbs and a pinch of garlic granules. Spread evenly on the pizza base.

2. Use the cheese recipe (from the pesto cups recipe in the next few pages of this book) and dollop this here and there on the pizza base.

3. Place a selection of finely chopped peppers, onions, mushrooms and anything else you fancy, on the tomato sauce and cheese base, and then place on a dehydrating tray at 104°F/40°C for 3-4 hours, until they look lightly cooked.

4. Eat warm from the dehydrator or cold later on.

5. I usually make twice the number of mini-bases that I need and then freeze them 'as is', to use for a quick meal at another time. They can be defrosted by popping into the dehydrator for 1-2 hours.

Raw Sausages

Ingredients

1½ to 2 carrots

200g chopped cabbage

125g ground sunflower seeds

2 tbsp. ground flaxseed

½ onion

1 tbsp. sesame seed oil

½ tsp of dried flaked seaweed

Directions

1. Add all ingredients to a food processor and process into a thick paste.

2. Shape into sausages and dehydrate at 104°F/40°C for 8-10 hours.

Raw Meatless Meatballs

Ingredients

150g sunflower seeds or pumpkin seeds

75g raw walnuts

150g sun-dried tomatoes (or half sun-dried and half fresh tomatoes)

1 tbsp. fresh lemon or lime juice

1 tbsp. sesame seed oil

½ tbsp. seaweed flakes

1-2 cloves garlic or 1-1½ tsp. garlic granules

¼ tsp. chopped basil or 1½ tsp. dried basil

1 tbsp. fresh minced rosemary or 1 tsp. dried

2 tbsp. fresh chopped oregano or ½ tsp. dried

½ tsp. chilli powder or cayenne pepper

½ small red onion, minced

Directions

1. Place the seeds and nuts in a bowl with enough fresh water to cover them and soak for 6-8 hours. Drain and rinse well. Do not allow to dry out before adding to the recipe.

2. Place sun-dried tomatoes (if not in oil) in a bowl with enough water to cover them and let soak for at least one hour. Drain off the water, save for later. Chop up tomatoes.

3. Place all ingredients into a food processor and blend until fine.

4. Form into small balls and place on greaseproof paper or waxed dehydrator sheets and place in dehydrator. Dehydrate for 1-2 hours at 104°F/40°C, remove from sheets and put straight onto the dehydrator tray for a further 10-12 hours (depending on size).

5. These freeze really well: you can make a double batch and freeze half for a later date. They can be defrosted by putting

them straight into the dehydrator from frozen and dehydrating them for around 2-3 hours. Eat them straight away!

Raw Pasta Sauce (Option 1)

Ingredients

6 tomatoes

1 avocado

3 carrots

2 sticks celery

8 dates

½ onion

2 tbsp. olive oil

2 tbsp. sesame seed oil

½ tsp. of dried flaked seaweed

4 tbsp. fresh basil

1 small garlic glove

¾ tsp. chilli powder or cayenne pepper

Directions

1. Roughly chop the tomatoes, avocado, carrots and celery. Put everything in a food processor and blend to a thick sauce.

2. Add this to the meatballs and spiralize some courgette, carrot and sweet potato pasta and you have a delicious, healthy, raw pasta dish.

Pasta Sauce (Option 2)

Ingredients

90g soaked cashews

180ml filtered water

1½ tsp. dried oregano or 3 tsp. fresh chopped oregano

1½ tsp. dried basil or 3 tsp. fresh chopped basil

1 tbsp. lemon or lime juice

1 tbsp. olive oil

¼ tbsp. garlic granules or one very small garlic clove

1 tsp. Himalayan salt

1 red pepper, chopped into small pieces (optional)

1 or 2 medium tomatoes, chopped into small pieces (optional)

Directions

1. Soak cashews for at least 2 hours, rinse well and then add to a food processor and blend until they form a batter-like mix.

2. Add all the other ingredients to the blender except the pepper and tomatoes.

3. Blend until it looks like a chunky sauce.

4. Add the sauce, the pepper and tomatoes to your pasta, mix well and place in the fridge for at least an hour, but preferably two.

Cheese and Pesto Boats

Ingredients for the Boats

8 medium cup-like mushrooms of your choice (or use baby peppers if you prefer, or go for a mix of both)

2 tbsp. olive oil

2 tbsp. lemon or lime juice (optional)

1 tbsp. sesame seed oil

½ tsp. dried flaked seaweed

¼ tsp. Himalayan salt

Directions

Rub all the above ingredients well into the mushrooms or peppers and leave to marinade for at least 2 hours.

Ingredients for the cheese mix

135g pine nuts that have been soaked for at least 2 hours

60ml filtered water

1 tbsp. lemon or lime juice

¼ tsp. Himalayan salt

Directions

Place all the ingredients into a food processor and blend until smooth.

Ingredients for the pesto

Either use the Wild Pesto recipe from this book, or this one:

60g fresh basil, chopped

60ml olive oil

¼ tsp. dried garlic granules or ½ small garlic clove

1 tsp. lemon or lime juice

50g walnuts soaked for at least 7 hours

¼ tsp. Himalayan salt

Directions

Place all ingredients in a food processor and blend until well mixed but still slightly lumpy.

To assemble cups

1. Place 1-2 tbsp. cheese into your mushroom or pepper
2. On top of this place 1 tsp. pesto
3. Place the cup onto a dehydrator tray and dehydrate at 104°F/40°C for 5-6 hours if using mushrooms. And for 104°F/40°C for 6-8 hours if using peppers.

Spinach Quiche

Ingredients for the base

380g chopped courgettes

60ml olive oil

1 tsp. ground almonds

120g ground flaxseed

Directions

1. Blend courgettes in a food processor until smooth.

2. Add remaining ingredients and blend again until well mixed.

Ingredients for the filling

190g white onion, chopped

1 tsp. sesame seed oil

½ tbsp. dried flaked seaweed

2 tsp. fresh garlic or 1 tsp. garlic granules

240g sunflower seeds

60ml lemon juice

120-150ml filtered water

500-600g well-packed, chopped spinach

1 tsp. sea salt

Directions

1. Put base batter into a quiche dish and spread evenly around bottom and sides.

2. Dehydrate at 104°F/40°C for 12-14 hours

3. Place onion pieces in a bowl with the sesame seed oil for at least 20 minutes.

4. Place all ingredients except the water and lemon juice into a high-speed blender and blend until well mixed. Add all remaining ingredients and blend until it has the consistency of cottage cheese.

5. Scoop filling onto the quiche base and dehydrate at 104**°F**/40**°C** for 4 hours.

6. Serve warm or cold

Garlic Oregano Crackers

Ingredients

75g flaxseeds

75g chia seeds

37g raw olive oil

110ml water (or more if needed)

1 medium tomato

1 tbsp. fresh oregano leaves chopped or 1 tbsp. dried

1 tbsp. mixed herbs

2 cloves garlic or 1 tsp. garlic granules

2 tbsp. fresh lime juice

1 tbsp. agave nectar, maple syrup or raw honey

½ tsp. Himalayan salt

½ tsp. onion powder

Pinch of pepper if you like, but not essential

Directions

1. Grind the flaxseeds and chia seeds into a powder and set to one side.
2. Blend all remaining ingredients in a high-speed blender, add seed powder and blend again.
3. Spread the batter on waxed dehydrator sheets or greaseproof paper.
4. Dehydrate for one hour at 104°F/40°C.
5. Turn thickened batter upside down and put straight onto dehydrator tray.
6. Lower temperature for 6-8 hours (depending on thickness) to 104°F/40°C.
7. Cut into cracker size and serve.

Juice Pulp Crackers

Ingredients

500g juice pulp

60g ground flaxseed

½ tsp. coriander

½ tsp. curry

1 tsp. sesame seed oil

½ tsp of dried flaked seaweed

1 tbsp. lemon juice

Directions

1. Mix all ingredients well, by hand or in a food processor. Add water if needed. I usually find that I don't need any (especially with cucumber and celery pulps, which are moist), but if you want the crackers to be less dense, go ahead and add 50 – 100ml of water to the mix. It should be malleable but still hold together.

2. Spread the mixture, about ¼ inch thick, to cover two to three dehydrator trays lined with a waxed dehydrator sheet.

3. Put into the dehydrator at 104°F/40°C for about 2 hours, then flip them onto the dehydrator tray. You can score the crackers at this point if you want. Dehydrate another 4-6 hours and there you have it.

4. If you don't have a dehydrator, bake these at 104°F/40°C in a conventional oven.

Kale Crisps

Ingredients

250g kale

1-2 tsp. olive oil (or sesame seed oil)

1 tsp. sea salt

1 tbsp. any other herbs or spices you like (optional)

Directions

1. Wash kale and pat dry.
2. Cut off any thick stems, slice leaves and place in a large bowl.
3. Add olive oil and salt.
4. Massage oil and salt into kale leaves.
5. Place kale on dehydrator trays (it will take up a lot of room until it wilts down).
6. Dehydrate at 104°F/40°C for 8-10 hours (or until crispy).
7. If you do not have a dehydrator, bake in a conventional oven on a low heat around 104°F/40°C for around 10 minutes (stir half way through).

Tip:

You can make vegetable crisps out of most vegetables. I like courgette, sweet potato and squash the best. Just slice thinly with a mandolin or a knife, or the slicing setting on a food processor and then follow the above instructions. Vegetables like these generally need twice as long in the dehydrator, as they are denser.

Avocado and Banana Chocolate Mousse

Ingredients

1 avocado, deseeded, peeled and sliced

1-2 bananas (depending on size)

4-6 tbsp. cacao powder

3-4 tbsp. agave nectar or honey

1 pinch of Himalayan or sea salt

Directions

1. Blend everything together in a food processor until smooth

2. Place into small bowls and freeze for 1-2 hours

3. Remove and serve as is or with a few berries on top

Gluten-free, Raw, Vegan Strawberry Cheesecake

Ingredients for the Base

30g desiccated coconut

300g chopped pecans

8-10 dates (soaked for a minimum of 1 hour)

Directions

1. Put all base ingredients into a food processor and process down.

2. Put mixture into a cake tin and pat down well.

Filling Ingredients

450g cashews, soaked (for at least 1 hour)

120g lemon juice

120g agave nectar, or maple syrup

80g melted coconut oil

¼ tsp. vanilla extract

380g chopped strawberries

Directions

1. Put all filling ingredients except the coconut oil into a blender and blend well.

2. Add the coconut oil and give it another quick blitz.

3. Pour filling mixture onto base mixture.

4. Add the chopped strawberries on top of the mixture.

5. Put the other cup of strawberries in the food processor and blend ever so slightly (so that you have both lumps and juice).

6. Pour this over the cheesecake.

7. 7. Leave to set for at least 2 hours in your fridge.

Raw Carrot Cake

Ingredients for the cake base

190g roughly chopped carrots

300g walnuts

200g raisins

60g shredded or desiccated coconut

4 tbsp. honey, agave nectar or maple syrup

2 tsp. vanilla extract

1 tsp. cinnamon

1-2 tsp. water

Icing ingredients

150g cashews

2 tbsp. lemon or lime juice

4 tbsp. honey, agave nectar or maple syrup

1 tsp. vanilla extract

1 tsp. water

Directions

1. Place carrots in food processor and process into small chunks. Add all the remaining cake base ingredients and process until everything is in small chunks but not a paste.
2. Place into a cake tin and pat down or use hands to mould into a cake shape if you do not have a cake tin.
3. Put all icing ingredients into the processor and process until a paste and ice the cake.
4. Put into fridge for a few hours to set.

Cookie Dough Balls

Ingredients

200g cashew nuts

200g of rolled oats

4 tbsp of cacao nibs

2 tsp of vanilla extract

6 tbsp of agave nectar

¼ tsp of ground sea or rock salt

Directions

1. Place cashews and oats into a food processor and blend until the mix looks like breadcrumbs

2. Add all the other ingredients until well mixed

3. Make mixture into small balls by pressing the mix tightly together in your hands

4. Place in the fridge for a minimum of 30 minutes to set and leave in the fridge when not eating them

Banana Balls

Ingredients

2 bananas, peeled

170g cashew nut butter (or a nut or seed butter of your choice)

150g dates, pitted

300g of walnuts, ground

1 tsp cinnamon

pinch of Himalayan or sea salt

Directions

1. Place all the ingredients in a blender and mix well.
2. The mixture should be a little sticky, if not, then add a little more nut butter, or if too sticky, add some more ground walnuts.
3. Roll mixture into balls with your hands and place on a plate.
4. Put balls into the fridge for a minimum of a couple of hours, but preferably overnight to harden slightly.
5. These beautiful balls freeze well too!

Sesame Seed Bars

Ingredients

300g sesame seeds

100g chia seeds

50g flax seeds, ground down

50g desiccated coconut

200g dried fruits, like raisins, sultanas, cranberries or goji berries

200g of tahini or other nut butter

60g of coconut oil, melted

80ml of agave nectar or maple syrup

10ml of vanilla extract

Pinch of Himalayan or sea salt

50 – 100g of cacao powder (depending how chocolatey you like it) – optional!

Directions

1. Place all the ingredients in a large mixing bowl and mix well.
2. If you want to make half the batch into chocolate flapjacks, then put half the mixture into another bowl and add the cacao and mix well.
3. Line baking trays with a liner of your choice and pour the mixture out and pat down well to create a firm flapjack-like mixture.
4. Place in the freezer for 2 hours and then remove and cut into portions and then return to the freezer until wanted. Remove an hour before eating or leave in the fridge overnight.

Fermented / Probiotic Foods

Probiotic: A substance which stimulates the growth of microorganisms, especially those with beneficial properties (such as those in the intestinal flora).

Up until not that long ago, much of our food was fermented. This preserved our food through the winter, when food was scarcer. Then chemically-laden preservatives came along and we, for the most part, got out of the habit of fermenting foods and drinks.

The consumption of regular amounts of fermented foods and drinks promotes good gut health. Please note that I do not mean pickled foods, as these carry a very minimal amount of goodness into the digestive system. By fermented, I mean cultured (food and drink traditionally made with a cultured starter) or lacto-fermented (traditionally made with salt and water). Both of these processes are highly nutritious. They are full of millions of beneficial yeasts and bacteria and are wonderfully detoxifying for the digestive system and thus the rest of the body.

Different types of fermented foods have slightly different strains of probiotics, so having a good range of these foods and drinks prepared in different ways is the most beneficial to your body. They can all be prepared at home and you can buy most of them from a good health food shop. When purchasing things like sauerkraut, kimchi or kombucha from a shop, check if they are unpasteurised. If they aren't, then they will have been heated in some way, their nutrients greatly diminished, and much of their goodness destroyed.

Why consume more fermented or cultured probiotic foods and drinks?

1. They restore the balance of the digestive system (the good yeasts and bacteria from the fermented foods and drinks literally attack the bad yeasts and bacteria in the digestive system).

2. They are high in enzymes, which help you to absorb and utilise the nutrients from your foods.

3. They promote better digestion of all foods and drinks, but especially foods that are typically hard to digest such as high fibre foods, grains, nuts, seeds and legumes (lentils, pulses, soy, etc.).

4. Many people who cannot tolerate dairy can actually tolerate fermented dairy items as the fermenting process breaks down the lactose in the food and drink.

5. Fermenting your own foods and drinks is really cheap, super-easy, and it means there is never a reason for any food to go to waste in your home ever again.

6. The fermented dairy items are particularly high in B vitamins.

7. Due to their balancing and detoxing effect, fermented foods can aid weight loss.

8. They also help balance out hormonal issues and strengthen the immune system.

9. They can help clear up skin concerns and promote healthy hair.

10. Many people find their general mood and energy levels improve.

SOME OF MY FAVOURITE FERMENT-ED FOOD AND DRINK RECIPES

Water Kefir

Kefir is an easy, yummy and extremely healthy fermented/cultured drink. You can do a second ferment with any flavour you wish. Anyone of any age can drink it. You will need to buy water kefir grains from an online source; there are lots of sellers on sites like eBay.

Ingredients

60g organic sugar

200ml hot water

720ml cold water

4 tbsp. water kefir grains

Directions

1. Put the sugar and hot water into a large Mason jar and allow to dissolve.
2. Then top up with cold water. (If the water is chlorinated, then leave aside for 24 hours to remove the chlorine before adding grains.)
3. Add the water kefir grains.
4. You can also add ½ tsp. of bicarbonate of soda, a squeeze of lemon, mineral drops or egg shell at this stage for added mineral content and healthy grains.
5. Secure some muslin or a coffee filter over the top of the Mason jar with a rubber band.
6. Let it culture for 2-3 days: a little shorter time if you prefer it sweet (with higher sugar content) and a little longer if you prefer it slightly more sour (lower sugar content).
7. When it reaches your preferred taste, use a plastic sieve (metal items can damage the grains) to separate the grains from the

liquid. Then put the grains directly into a new batch of sugar water (as above) to start a new batch.

8. You can now drink the liquid as it is, but make sure to store it in the fridge to prevent further fermentation.

9. Or you can now do a second ferment to add more flavour and fizz to your kefir. Add juiced fruit, or even vegetables like beetroot, to the kefir drink and put in a Mason jar or swing-top Grolsch-style bottle and close the lid firmly. This will allow the kefir to get fizzy like a flavoured soda. Leave this for another 24-72 hours and then store in the fridge when it is at your preferred taste.

Helpful Hints:

1. Do not rinse grains in normal water if they need rinsing: use sugar water or coconut water.

2. Boil egg shells before using: if you don't, they can cause mould.

3. In my opinion, your fruit drink will taste much better if you juice the fruit, rather than adding in just whole pieces. If you add whole pieces, they will need straining off.

4. Your grains should multiply with each batch. If this is not happening, then you may need to add more sugar or minerals as this generally means your grains aren't happy.

5. Sweet fruits generally work better than sour fruits, especially strawberries: yum!

6. I mention again: don't use metal utensils (including sieves) with the grains as this can harm them.

7. If you buy dehydrated grains, you may need to go through a few batches to get them going properly. Be patient!

8. If you don't want to make another batch straight away, then put your grains into some super sugary water in the fridge (making sure to add more sugar after a week or so).

9. Eventually, you'll have too many grains. Why not give the extra ones to a friend, so that they can start fermenting their own kefir. You can even eat the excess kefir grains!

Milk Kefir

Ingredients

900ml raw milk (or organic whole milk)

1-2 tbsp. milk kefir grains (these are not the same grains as water kefir ones, but can be purchased from the same sites).

Directions

1. Place your kefir grains in the Mason jar and add the milk.

2. Stir with a wooden spoon (remember, no metal as this can harm the grains), cover and secure with muslin and elastic band and leave at room temperature to culture for up to 1-3 days, depending on preferred taste or room temperature.

3. A shorter fermentation time will mean a milder flavour and a longer one will mean a stronger and sourer flavour.

4. Once your kefir is done culturing, remove the grains (this is usually easier with your hands as it can be quite thick). Store the kefir milk in the refrigerator and begin another batch with the grains.

Kombucha

Kombucha is a fermented tea drink that, when left to a second ferment, gets really fizzy and can resemble champagne. It's delicious, especially if you use a flavoured green tea like jasmine, as I do. You will need to order the scoby / mushroom / mother online which will come in a small amount of kombucha tea with which to start off your first batch.

Ingredients

800ml tea (cooled)

3 tbsp. organic sugar

one scoby / mushroom / mother in 200ml of kombucha tea

Directions

1. Pour 800ml of boiling water over a teabag in a large Mason jar and add 3-4 tbsp. sugar.
2. Allow to brew for 10-20 minutes and then remove the tea bag.
3. Cool to room temperature.
4. Add your scoby and 200ml of a previous batch of kombucha tea to the jar.
5. Cover the top of the jar securely with some muslin or a coffee filter and an elastic band.
6. Place the jar in a cool place away from direct sunlight, such as in a cupboard.
7. Let your kombucha brew for 7-10 days (depending if you prefer yours slightly sweeter or slightly more sour), but note that the less time you leave it, the more sugar and caffeine it will contain.
8. Another kombucha scoby (a baby) will grow during this time. Use this to make a second batch, give it away or cut it into small squares, dehydrate them and eat as a treat.

9. After 7-10 days, pour about 500ml of your brewed kombucha out of your jar, sieve and it's ready to drink (make sure to store in your fridge). Remove the baby scoby at this point also.

10. Replace the kombucha you have just poured out with a new batch of sugared tea and leave to sit as above. This is the procedure to follow for each batch.

11. Second fermentation: after sieving the kombucha tea, add a fruit of your choice (either juiced down or chopped up), bottle it, cap it tightly and leave to sit for a further 2-4 days in the fridge. The end result should be a bubbly, champagne-like, refreshing drink. If it does not get fizzy, this is usually because there is not enough sugar in the drink for the process to work.

Note:

· The longer kombucha tea brews, the more vinegary it becomes.
· Every time you make a new batch of kombucha tea, a new baby scoby is formed.
· Avoid artificial sweeteners and honey while fermenting kombucha tea.

Beet Kvass

Ingredients

2-4 fresh beetroots

40-60ml juice from sauerkraut

1 tbsp. sea salt or Himalayan salt

Filtered water (to cover)

Directions

1. Wash beets and peel if not organic; leave skin on if organic.

2. Chop beets into small cubes: don't grate.

3. Place beets in Mason jar.

4. Add sauerkraut juice and salt. (If you don't want to use sauerkraut juice, double the salt. It may take longer to ferment.)

5. Fill jar with filtered water.

6. Cover with muslin and leave on the counter at room temperature for 2 days to ferment.

7. Transfer to fridge.

Apple Cider Vinegar

Ingredients

6-10 organic apples (whole or scraps of)

water (to fill your chosen Mason jar)

Directions

1. Rinse apples/scraps and cut into large chunks.
2. Put the apples in a bowl and cover with the muslin and allow to go brown (which should take no longer than an hour).
3. When sufficiently brown, put apples into the jar and cover with water.
4. Cover the jar with the muslin and leave in a dark place for 2-4 months (shorter time for scraps and longer for larger chunks of apple).
5. Strain and discard the apple pieces and any scum from the liquid, and bottle the vinegar in an airtight container. Use as and when required.

Sauerkraut

Ingredients

1 medium cabbage

1 tbsp. sea salt

Optional:

1 tbsp. caraway, coriander or fennel seeds

3 tbsp. grated ginger (I highly recommend this addition)

200 – 300g grated carrot

Directions

1. Remove outer leaves from the cabbage and set them aside.
2. Shred cabbage. I like to use the grating option of my food processor for this.
3. Shred carrots and ginger (if you're adding these).
4. In a bowl, mix the shredded items with seeds (if you're adding these) and sea salt, then massage together or pound down with a mallet or the end of a rolling pin for 10 minutes.
5. Once the juices have been released, place into a wide-mouthed jar and continue to pound down until juices come up and cover the cabbage. (If this does not happen, then add a little fresh water until it covers the cabbage well.) Leave a space of 2 inches at the top.
6. Place a whole cabbage leaf over the top of the shredded cabbage, making sure no air can get to the cabbage underneath. If you have no cabbage leaf, then use a clean weight of some sort to weigh it down.
7. Leave in a dark place at room temperature for around a month. You can eat it after 3 days, but it's much tastier and contains more probiotics if left longer. Transfer to fridge once you open it or after a month or two.

If you leave it to sit for more than a couple of weeks, you may want to 'burp' it (open the lid a little) to release the built-up pressure from the jar.

Celeriac and Ginger Kraut

Ingredients

1 celeriac, peeled and chopped into quarters

2-3 cms of fresh ginger

1 tsp. mustard or coriander seeds

2 tsp. Himalayan or sea salt

Directions

1. Using the grating/shredding function on a food processor, grate the celeriac and ginger and add to a large bowl with the salt and spices and mix well.

2. Squeeze the juice from the vegetables and then pack everything (including the juice) into a few jars.

3. Make sure everything is below the level of the juice, if it is not, add a little extra water until it is.

4. Make sure there is at least 2 cms of space in the top of the jars.

5. Cut the cabbage leaf into a slightly bigger shape than the jar and tuck it down around the edge of the kraut mixture in the jar, making sure everything, including the leaf is below the juice/brine level. If you have no cabbage leaf, then use a clean weight of some sort to weigh it down and place lid on jar.

6. Burp/let the gas out every day (or twice daily if it seems lively) until it stops gassing.

7. Once it stops gassing, it is ready to consume. Once you start consuming from the jar, keep it in the fridge.

Beetroot and Ginger Kraut

Ingredients

4-5 large beetroot, washed, top and tailed

½ a small red cabbage

5-6 cms of fresh ginger

2 tsp. Himalayan or sea salt

Directions

1. Using the grating/shredding function on a food processor, grate the beetroot, cabbage and ginger and add to a large bowl with the salt and mix well.

2. Squeeze the juice from the vegetables and then pack everything (including the juice) into a few jars.

3. Make sure everything is below the level of the juice, if it is not, add a little extra water until it is.

4. Make sure there is at least 2 cms of space in the top of the jars.

5. Cut the cabbage leaf into a slightly bigger shape than the jar and tuck it down around the edge of the kraut mixture in the jar, making sure everything, including the leaf is below the juice/brine level. If you have no cabbage leaf, then use a clean weight of some sort to weigh it down and place lid on jar.

6. Burp/let the gas out every day (or twice daily if it seems lively) until it stops gassing.

7. Once it stops gassing, it is ready to consume. Once you start consuming from the jar, keep it in the fridge.

Curried Squash Kraut

Ingredients

1 smashed squash, de-seeded and peeled

4 large carrots

1 tsp. ginger granules or 2-3 cms of fresh ginger

1 tsp. garlic granules or 1 clove garlic, mashed

1 tbsp. of curry powder

1 tsp. cumin seeds

1 tsp. mustard seeds

3 tsp. Himalayan salt

Directions

1. Using the grating/shredding function in the food processor grate the squash, carrots and ginger.

2. Place these and all the other ingredients in a bowl and mix well.

3. Squeeze the juice from the vegetables and then pack everything (including the juice) into a few jars.

4. Make sure everything is below the level of the juice, if it is not, add a little extra water until it is.

5. Make sure there is at least 2 cms of space in the top of the jars.

6. Cut the cabbage leaf into a slightly bigger shape than the jar and tuck it down around the edge of the kraut mixture in the jar, making sure everything, including the leaf is below the juice/brine level. If you have no cabbage leaf, then use a clean weight of some sort to weigh it down and place lid on jar.

7. Burp/let the gas out every day (or twice daily if it seems lively) until it stops gassing.

8. Once it stops gassing it is ready to consume. Once you start consuming from the jar, keep it in the fridge.

Indian Cabbage and Carrot Kraut

Ingredients

1 small white cabbage

1 small yellow onion

3 garlic cloves

4 cms of ginger, peeled

½ tsp. cumin seeds

½ tsp. mustard seeds

½ tsp. coriander seeds

½ tsp. fennel seeds

½ tsp. black peppercorns

½ tsp. turmeric powder

1 tsp. curry powder

1 tsp. Himalayan or sea salt

Directions

1. Place cabbage, carrots, onion, garlic and ginger in a food processor using the grating/shredding function

2. Put all the ingredients in a bowl and mix well and start squeezing/massaging or pounding to release all the liquid from the ingredients.

3. Place into a medium jar and pack down, then fill with filtered water.

4. Make sure everything is below the level of the water, if it is not, add a little extra water until it is.

5. Make sure there is at least 2 cms of space in the top of the jars.

6. Cut the cabbage leaf into a slightly bigger shape than the jar and tuck it down around the edge of the kraut mixture in the jar, making sure everything, including the leaf is below the juice/

brine level. If you have no cabbage leaf, then use a clean weight of some sort to weigh it down and place lid on jar.

7. Burp/let the gas out every day (or twice daily if it seems lively) until it stops gassing.
8. Once it stops gassing, it is ready to consume. Once you start consuming from the jar, keep it in the fridge.

Christmas Kraut

Ingredients

½ large white cabbage

3 apples

2 tsp. cloves

1 tsp. cinnamon

½ tsp. nutmeg

½ tsp. mixed spice

1 tsp. of Himalayan salt

Directions

1. Using a food processor on the shredding/grating function, grate the cabbage and apples. Save the outer leaf of the cabbage.

2. Add to a large bowl with all the other ingredients and mix well.

3. Squeeze the juice/brine from the cabbage and apples.

4. Add everything, including the juice/brine, into a sterilised jar and pack down well.

5. Make sure there is at least a 2cm gap at the top of the jar.

6. Add more water if the juice/brine does not come above the kraut mixture.

7. Cut the cabbage leaf into a slightly bigger shape than the jar and tuck it down around the edge of the kraut mixture in the jar, making sure everything, including the leaf, is below the juice/brine level. If you have no cabbage leaf, then use a clean weight of some sort to weigh it down and place lid on jar.

8. Clear all the bits off the inside of the jar and put the lid on.

9. Burp/open the jar every day for the first week to allow the gases to escape (this is very important).

10. Consume once gassing has stopped (around a week) and place in fridge once you start eating from the jar.

Miso Kimchi

Ingredients

½ a large cabbage, chopped into inch squares

1 red pepper, chopped into inch squares

1 yellow pepper, chopped into inch squares

1 bag of radishes, sliced

1 bunch of spring onions, chopped

2 leeks, cut length-ways and then chopped

2 inches of ginger, grated

2 garlic cloves, grated

4-6 tsp. of chilli powder (more if you prefer it hotter)

4 tbsp. of miso paste

3 tsp. of Himalayan or sea salt

2 tbsp. of seaweed flakes (optional, but to my mind, highly desirable for taste and nutrient content)

Directions

1. Chop everything as directed above and add to a large bowl
2. Add the salt and seaweed and mix well, cover and leave for 30 minutes
3. Stir well, cover and leave for another 30 minutes
4. Stir well once again, cover and leave for another 30 minutes
5. Add the miso paste a little at a time and mix really well
6. Add the chilli powder and again mix well
7. Add all the ingredients to a large Mason jar (or a couple of smaller ones)
8. Pack down tightly and add a little fresh water to fill up any air gaps
9. Weigh everything down under the water level (making sure there is at least 2 cm air gap at the top of the jar)

10. Leave to one side in your kitchen (not in direct sunlight) for a minimum of 5 days (I prefer twice this time for a stronger kimchi)

11. Make sure to burp (open the jars) each day to release any gases that will build up

12. Place in a fridge and start consuming when ready

Chunky Carrot and Radish Kimchi

Ingredients

2 carrots, thinly sliced

1 bunch of radishes, topped, tailed and quartered

½ a bunch of spring onions, chopped

2-3 cms of fresh ginger, thinly sliced

3-4 garlic cloves, thinly sliced

2 tbsp. sesame seed oil

2 tbsp. of dried seaweed

1 tsp. chilli powder

1 tsp. black pepper, freshly ground

1 tsp. Himalayan or sea salt

Directions

- Place all the ingredients in a bowl and mix well.
- Place into a medium jar and pack down, then fill with filtered water.
- Make sure everything is below the level of the water, if it is not, add a little extra water until it is.
- Make sure there is at least 2 cms of space in the top of the jars.
- Weigh everything down with a cabbage leaf, a pebble or a kitchen weight of some description.
- Burp/let the gas out every day (or twice daily if it seems lively) until to stops gassing.
- Once it stops gassing, it is ready to consume. Once you start consuming from the jar, put it in the fridge.

Kimchi Kraut

Ingredients

½ head white cabbage

2 carrots (parsnips also work well)

7-8 red radishes

1 small celeriac (optional)

1 small yellow onion

2-inch square fresh ginger

4 cloves garlic (optional)

1 tsp. dried chilli flakes

1 tbsp. salt

25-50ml filtered water or sauerkraut juice

Directions

1. Using the shredding/grating function on your food processor, or a hand grater, grate all the vegetables.
2. Place all ingredients except the water into a large bowl and massage the salt thoroughly through the vegetables.
3. Using either a kraut pounder or the end of a rolling pin, pound down the vegetables until the juices are released. This should take around 10-15 minutes. You can also squeeze the juice from the veggies with your hands, which is sometimes easier on the arms.
4. Put the vegetable mixture into the jars.
5. If the brine mixture from the vegetables does not completely cover them, then top up with water until it does.
6. Put a couple of cabbage leaves on the top of your vegetable mixture and weigh down with a clean, boiled stone or a kitchen weight. Make sure everything is just under the water/brine level, so that it does not go mouldy.

7. Put the lid on the jar and place in a cupboard for a minimum of 2 weeks, preferably a month. The longer you leave it the better, but if you leave it longer than 6 weeks you will need to 'burp' the jar. It will taste stronger, the longer you leave it.

8. Once opened, put in the fridge. Use it as a side to just about any hot or cold dish for a super-charged meal.

Note:

You can use just about any vegetables in this recipe, so it's a great way to use up left over veggies!

Sourdough Bread

Ingredients

480g flour (I prefer spelt flour)

100g sourdough starter

220ml fresh water

1 tsp. salt

1 tsp. sugar

Directions

1. In a bowl, mix well 100g of sourdough starter with 300g of flour and 220ml of water and cover for 8-10 hours. (At this or any of the later stages you can add herbs, chillies, sundried tomatoes or other similar items).

2. Add the remaining 180g of flour, the sugar and salt, and knead well. Cover and allow to rest for another 2-3 hours.

3. Knead again and pop into a lightly oiled bread tin or proof basket, cover, and leave in a warm place for 1-2 hours. (You can lightly score the top of the dough at this stage if you want to.)

4. Preheat your oven on a medium heat (around 350°F/180°C/gas mark 4) and put a bowl of boiling water on the bottom of your oven.

5. Place dough in its baking tin/baking basket in the upper part of the oven and bake for 30-35 minutes.

6. Remove from the tin and allow it to cool slightly before cutting into it.

Notes:

* Your sourdough starter needs to be fed once a week and should live in your fridge until the day before you want to use it.

* To feed your sourdough starter, add 50g flour and 50ml fresh water. Mix well and pop back in the fridge until you want to use it.

* Your starter will separate (with the hooch lying on top). This is absolutely fine, and it just needs stirring back in each week when you feed it.

Fermented Salsa

Ingredients

6 tomatoes, chopped

2 red onions, chopped

3 red, yellow and/or green peppers, chopped

4-5 spring onions, chopped

2-3 medium chillis, finely sliced

3 garlic cloves, minced

1-2 limes, just the juice

1 tsp. cayenne pepper, ground

1 tsp. paprika, ground

2 tsp. Himalayan or sea salt

Directions

1. Place everything in a large jar and squash it all down.
2. Add filtered water to cover the vegetables.
3. Make sure everything is below the level of the water.
4. Make sure there is at least 2 cms of space in the top of the jars.
5. Weigh everything down with a clean, boiled pebble, a kitchen weight or a bag full of water.
6. Burp/let the gas out every day (or twice daily if it seems lively) until it stops gassing.
7. Once it stops gassing it is ready to consume.
8. Once you start consuming from the jar, keep it in the fridge.

Pineapple and Papaya Salsa

Ingredients

1 small pineapple, peeled and chopped into small pieces

2 papayas, peeled, de-seeded and chopped into small pieces

1 medium red onion, peeled and chopped into small pieces

1 large pepper (colour of your choosing), de-seeded and chopped into small pieces

4-6 inches of fresh ginger, peeled and diced or grated into tiny pieces

1-3 fresh chillis (depending how hot you like it), cut into very small pieces

1 bunch of parsley, finely chopped

1-2 tsp. of garlic granules

1-2 tbsp. of the juice of an already fermented sauerkraut or kimchi

1 tbsp of ground Himalayan or sea salt

1-2 tsp chilli powder (optional)

Directions

1. Add all the ingredients to a large bowl and mix well.
2. Place into two medium jars and pack down, then fill with filtered water.
3. Make sure everything is below the level of the water.
4. Make sure there is at least 2 cms of space in the top of the jars.
5. Weigh everything down with a cabbage leaf, a pebble or a kitchen weight of some description.
6. Burp/let the gas out every day (or twice daily if it seems lively) until to stops gassing.
7. This is ready after 3 days, but I prefer to leave it 5 days for extra probiotic-ness. Once you start consuming from the jar, put it in the fridge.

Onion Relish

Ingredients

3 or 4 large onions, peeled and sliced thinly or grated

1-2 tbsp. peppercorns

2 tsp. Himalayan or sea salt

Filtered water, to cover

Directions

1. Place all the dry ingredients in a large bowl and mix well.
2. Leave covered for 30 minutes, until some of the liquid from the onions is starting to collect in the bowl.
3. Place everything (including the liquid) into a Mason jar and press down so that the liquid comes up above the onions. Add a little filtered water if this does not happen.
4. Place the lid firmly on the jar.
5. 'Burp' or release the gas from the jar every day for the first week and then weekly after that.
6. The relish is ready to eat after a week and for many months thereafter.

Spicy Fermented Aubergine Dip

Ingredients

1 large aubergine

4-6 garlic cloves, diced

1 tsp. chilli flakes

½ tsp. paprika

1-2 tsp. dried basil

1-2 tsp. dried coriander

½ pepper, freshly ground

½ tsp. Himalayan sea salt (depending on size of aubergine)

Optional: 6-8 sun-dried tomatoes (in oil), chopped

Directions

1. Cut the aubergine up into squares and add to a large bowl with the salt and mix well.

2. Leave to sit for an hour or two (stir half way through) with some muslin or a tea-towel over the top.

3. Place all the other ingredients in the bowl with the aubergine and mix well. If it is not all mushy, then use a fork to mash it all down into more of a dip consistency.

4. Pack it all down into a jar (including the liquid from inside the aubergine) and if the liquid does not come above the aubergine mix, then add a little filtered water until it does.

5. Make sure there is at least 2 cms of space in the top of the jar and then place the lid on top.

6. Burp or let the gas out every day (or twice daily if it seems lively) until it stops gassing.

7. Once it stops gassing it is ready to consume. Once you start consuming from the jar, keep it in the fridge.

Fermented Mango Chutney

Ingredients

2 small mangoes, peeled, de-seeded and chopped

1 small red onion, finely chopped

4 cms of fresh ginger, peeled and finely chopped

1 garlic clove, peeled and minced

1 tsp. chilli flakes

½ tsp. curry powder

2 tbsp. sauerkraut, kimchi or other fermenting juice (I like to use fermented salsa juice)

1 tsp. Himalayan or sea salt

juice of 1 lime

Directions

1. Place all the ingredients in a bowl and mix well.
2. Pack it all down into a jar and if the liquid does not come above the mango mixture then add a little filtered water until it does.
3. Weigh down with a kitchen weight or pebble, to make sure everything is below the level of the water.
4. Make sure there is at least 2 cms of space in the top of the jar and then place the lid on top.
5. Burp/let the gas out every day (or twice daily if it seems lively) until it stops gassing.
6. Once it stops gassing, it is ready to consume. Once you start consuming from the jar, store it in the fridge.

Fermented Vegan 'Cheese'

Ingredients

300g cashews, soaked overnight

1 bunch of chives, chopped thinly

1 garlic clove, minced or ½ a tsp. of garlic granules

½ tsp. pepper freshly ground

Juice of 1 lemon

2 tsbp. of sauerkraut or kimchi juice (if you want a little spice)

1 tsp. raw apple cider vinegar

50-100ml of filtered water (start with 50 and add a little at a time until it's a little runny)

1 tsp. of Himalyan or sea salt

Directions

1. Rinse off soaked cashews.
2. Place all the ingredients apart from the chives into a food processor and blend well.
3. If the mixture isn't slightly runny (but not watery) then add a little more water until it is.
4. Place the mixture in a bowl and add the chives and mix well.
5. Cover the bowl with a tea-towel or muslin and an elastic band and leave on the kitchen side overnight.
6. Place into a medium-sized jar and leave in the fridge for up to two weeks.

Wild Garlic Pesto

Ingredients

700g-1kg wild garlic leaves

120g pine nuts or chopped almonds

1 tbsp. salt

60ml filtered water

50-100g basil leaves

salt and pepper

Directions

1. Blend all the ingredients except the water in a food processor. (You can change the ratio of ingredients to your personal taste.)

2. Add mixture to a jar and top up with the water so it comes just above the level of the mixture.

3. Place a small plate or weight over the top of the mixture so that it is all submerged.

4. Pop the lid onto the jar and put in a cupboard for anywhere between 10 days and 2 months. Place in the fridge once opened.

Helpful Hints:

- You can ferment the wild garlic by itself (as per the above directions), so that you have a store of probiotic garlic to last you through the winter.

- You can add olive oil to the jar rather than brine/salted water and this will make a pesto closer to shop-bought pesto and one that you can use almost straight away.

- Don't pull up the wild garlic bulbs – the leaves (and flowers) are the best bit of wild garlic and if you leave the bulbs in place, even more wild garlic will be there next year.

More Helpful Hints

❧ If you're not very healthy, have digestive issues, eat a lot of sugar, or suspect that you have a yeast overgrowth, then you should have only a small amount of any probiotic food or drink each day and slowly increase your intake. If you consume too much to start with, you may experience strong detox symptoms. These symptoms can be very unpleasant. If you find your tummy is churning a little bit, this is fine, but anything more than this means you're taking too much, too quickly.

❧ Although the little probiotic drinks, yogurts and pills you can buy in the shops do indeed contain beneficial probiotics, they have only a tiny fraction of the amount contained in fermented foods and drinks. Also, many of these items have additional sugars, sweeteners and nasty fillers in their ingredients list.

❧ Don't get hung up on exact measurements and timings with raw and fermented foods and drinks. They will taste delicious and be extremely good for you, no matter what. If you don't have the exact ingredients or leave something fermenting or dehydrating a little longer than recommended in my recipes, it really doesn't matter. It's better to do something than nothing at all, so give it a go and see how you get on.

* If your kitchen (or wherever you are placing your ferments) is hot, then the above processes will happen faster. If, on the other hand, it is cold, they will happen much slower.

* You can ferment most vegetables you come across. Firmer vegetables tend to do better in a kraut or kimchi sort of ferment, and softer vegetables tend to do better whole or in larger slices. Whatever kinds of veggies you choose, just make sure to pack them into the jar tightly and ensure they don't rise above the brine; otherwise they will go mouldy.

* If you find your fermented vegetables aren't very crisp, then you may want to consider adding an olive leaf or a raspberry leaf or two to the ferment. These will keep them crisp.

* If you have an issue with histamines, then you would want to address this before starting on fermented foods and drinks, as they are high histamine producers.

Resources

Raw Food – **Ani Phyo**

Easy Raw Vegan Dehydrating – **Kristen Suzanne**

Eat Smart Eat Raw: Detox Recipes for a High-Energy Diet – **Kate Wood**

Cultured Food for Life – **Donna Schwenk**

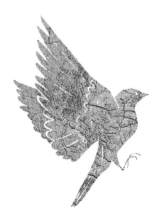

CHAPTER 9

THE LITTLE CRITTERS

*Our body teaches us that health lies in balance and harmony, rather than in conflict and fighting – **Ilchi Lee***

S tudies have shown that around 70% of us have a fungal imbalance and/or a parasite issue in our digestive system. (Other names for a fungus imbalance are: candida, thrush, athlete's foot, fungal infestation, bacterial imbalance and yeast overgrowth). Fungal issues develop over a period of time, and are caused by long-term stress, bad eating and drinking habits, drug use (both legal and illegal), antibiotics, steroids, oral contraceptive medication or a combination of any of the above.

As the ecology of your digestive system starts to break down, bad yeasts and bacteria start to take hold. Your digestive system also becomes a lovely inviting home to parasites. Initially, you may not notice any symptoms or side effects of this, but eventually, sometimes years later, you may notice your health isn't quite right, that that 'Monday morning feeling' never goes away, and that you may also have started to have some of the symptoms below, or even most of them.

1. flu / sinus problems / coughs / sore throats

2. IBS / upset tummy / constipation / indigestion

3. depression

4. PMS / mood swings / irritability

5. headaches / migraines

6. chronic fatigue / low energy levels

7. inability to lose weight / weight gain

8. itchy skin

9. poor concentration / feeling generally muddled

10. skin conditions / acne / eczema

11. dizziness

12. muscle weakness / pain

13. food and chemical sensitivity

14. low libido

15. thrush / athlete's foot

16. poor absorption of nutrients

The reason for this is because as the fungus grows, it produces toxins that spread throughout the body. They can affect all areas of the body and especially run amok through the digestive and endocrine systems, potentially affecting your hormones, thyroid function and insulin production. The more the fungus grows, the more toxins it produces, and the more overrun the body becomes. Your body works hard to try to remove these toxins and at the same time, the fungus is producing more and more of them. Without some additional help, the body simply cannot deal with the fungus and its friends, the parasites, and your health steadily goes downhill.

The good news is that it is fairly easy to bring the fungus back into normal healthy balance. You can do this in one (or a combination) of the following ways.

Detoxing the body

If you create an environment in your body that the fungus and parasites do not like, they will leave. If you follow the recommendations in this book, eventually your digestive system will become balanced again. You can help your body do this by cutting out processed foods, sugars and alcohol, and consuming a combination of detoxing herbs.

These three herbs are especially powerful at eliminating fungus and parasites: **wormwood, black walnut and clove**. However, if you are in any doubt, see a qualified herbalist who will advise you on how and when to take these and any others. You can also introduce anti-candida foods into your diet, such as **ginger, garlic** and **coconut oil.**

Fermented Foods and Drinks

As mentioned in the previous chapter, because fermented foods and drinks are full of good bacteria, yeasts and probiotics, when you consume these, they help to rebalance the digestive system, eliminate the overgrowth of fungus and eventually encourage the parasites to leave.

Try to have as many different strains (different fermented foods and drinks) as possible for optimum benefits. Start with a very small amount each day, maybe a tablespoonful, and slowly build up; otherwise you may find you have some pretty bad side effects as the fermented foods and drinks efficiently detox the digestive system. A slight churning of the stomach is a good sign: it means the good stuff in the fermented produce is attacking the bad stuff in your gut. However, if you have any symptoms worse than this, please reduce your consumption and slowly build it up again.

Zappers

Zappers are wonderful little health aids. A traditional zapper looks like a small box that has two electrodes and a strap attached to it. You wear it next to your skin (on the lowest setting to start with, and never above 12 volts) for 60 minutes in the morning, afternoon and evening (a total of 3 hours). It literally draws toxins out, right through the skin. It also kills many viruses, bacteria, fungus and parasites in the body. It also helps to ground you and reduces the effects of electromagnetic stress, because it is negatively charged, just like our planet. Zappers help alkalise and balance the body and they remove everything from herpes and Lyme disease to emotional blockages throughout the body. These are not recommended for anyone who has a pacemaker or is pregnant.

Enemas and Colonics

Enemas and colonics are very effective at removing those pesky critters from the digestive system. Enemas are fairly easy to do at home, but in my opinion they don't get high enough up the digestive tract to completely remove all the fungus and parasites. Colonics, however, do. I highly recommend going to a fully qualified colonic expert, preferably with a medical or nutritional background. They will be able to tell you if you have a fungus and/or parasite issue and recommend the best course of action to help support the treatments they give you. (Multiple treatments are necessary for effectiveness.)

Yeast Die-off Diet

This option is a bit more drastic, but effective. There are many die-off diets around, some lasting years, some just a few days, some using pills and potions, and some not. The die-off diet I recommend lasts around three weeks (slightly less for moderate cases and slightly more for severe cases).

A die-off diet aims at starving the fungus so that it returns to a healthy level in the body. To do this, you need to completely cut out all **sugars**; this includes fruit sugars, milk sugars and honey, as well as all the bad sugars. You also need to cut out all **yeasts** and **funguses** and this includes mushrooms, vinegars, blue cheeses, pickled goods and alcohol. On top of this, you need to cut out **all items that create a sugary / yeasty effect** in the body, so this includes all **refined carbohydrates**, and many white foods like white potatoes, white flour, pasta and white rice.

Tomatoes and carrots are both fine raw but when cooked they become sugary, so they are best avoided or dramatically cut down during this period.

You should try, whenever possible, to only eat **organic** foods, especially where meat and dairy are concerned. These two types of foods, if not organic, contain a high number of antibiotics and added hormones that fungus loves. Any pesticides and preservatives on fruits and veggies are a little gold mine for the fungus also, so if you can't manage organic, make sure you wash pesticides off shop-bought items well.

If you are sensitive to any particular foods or chemicals, then these need to be avoided during your diet to help the body heal and the immune system to strengthen.

During this time of change, it is very important to have a varied and balanced diet. Varying your diet will minimise food sensitivities and help your digestive system work more effectively, as well as give you a good supply of essential nutrients.

Anything you can do to strengthen the immune system is going to help, so make sure you have adequate amounts of **vitamin C, zinc** and **selenium**.

Drink at least **2-3 litres of water** per day to flush out the fungus and its toxins and to support a healthy digestive tract. You can make this water more alkaline by adding cucumber, ginger or pH drops.

Cut out, or at least cut down, caffeinated drinks, and replace them with **herbal teas,** especially ones that support the liver, like nettle and dandelion.

Make sure to take a **daily probiotic**, (if you are not consuming fermented foods and drinks), one with many millions of strains of lactobacillus bacteria.

Grapefruit seed extract (not grapeseed extract) is highly recommended. Please read the label, consume only as advised, and start with the minimum dose. This is a very strong, natural antifungal and isn't for everyone, so if you find this is too much for you, then please discontinue use. This is also not advised over the long term.

Oregano oil extract is an excellent natural antifungal, but again it is fairly strong, so it shouldn't be taken long term. And although it suggests on the label that you can put this, undiluted, directly into your mouth, I would not recommend this unless you want to be hopping about the kitchen trying to scrape the taste off your tongue for the next hour (as I was).

I would not recommend taking the above antifungals for longer than 12 weeks, which is the usual amount of time it takes for all the toxins from the fungus to leave the body after a die-off diet.

Lastly, try having daily **Epsom salt baths** to help draw out the toxins created by the fungus and the die-off diet itself.

You will likely be feeling under the weather during this time, and you will know when the die-off is finished when, literally, you wake up one morning (usually around the 3-week mark) feeling absolutely fine again.

I talk about this type of cleanse in far more detail in my book **Cleanse – The Holistic Detox Program for Mind, Body & Soul.**

Resources

*Cleanse – The Holistic Detox Program for Mind, Body & Soul – **Faith Canter***

*The Body Ecology Diet - **Donna Gates***

*Candida Albicans - **Leon Chaitow***

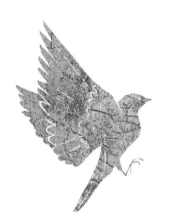

CHAPTER 10

DOES EATING ORGANIC
REALLY MAKE A DIFFERENCE?

When God created the Garden of Eden, She didn't use synthetic fertilizers, pesticides, herbicides and GMO apples – **Khang Kijarro Nguyen**

With so many conflicting reports out there, it is often hard to know what to do when it comes to organic food. I think we all know deep down, that the chemicals and pesticides sprayed onto our food and onto the soil it grows in can't be very good for us. But does it really make a difference? Would our health really improve if we only ate organic produce?

Up until the 1950s, all food was organic, there were no chemical pesticides, fertilisers or preservatives. Food was highly nutritious, locally sourced, fresh and tasty. What changed was the invention of these chemical fertilisers and preservatives. It meant that farmers could produce larger crops, ship them longer distances and reduce wastage caused by pest infestations.

However, many now believe that using these chemical pesticides caused more problems than it solved. It soon became apparent that these chemicals destroyed more than the odd pest. They also destroyed the natural ecosystem of the soil in which we grow our food. The micronutrients that were present in the soil soon began to disappear and today, our foods have become depleted in essential nutrients and enzymes, making them less tasty, not so fresh and not so good for us.

The problem is so bad now that many of our foods are fortified with laboratory-produced nutrients to try and ensure we get what our bodies require. For instance, today, cattle are injected with vitamin B12 as there is no longer enough of this in the soil to filter through the grass the cattle eat, the cattle themselves and then to us.

If we then add on the toxic effects of the chemicals our food produce is laced with, we end up with food that isn't all that healthy and could potentially cause health issues.

The toxic chemicals found in our food can cause health concerns ranging from headaches and skin conditions to chemical and food sensitivities. They may also cause poor gut health, fatigue, weight gain, some forms of depression, learning difficulties and increase our risk of some forms of cancer and autoimmune conditions.

While it's true that organic food is also no longer as nutrient-dense as it once was, as soils, for the most part, simply do not hold what they once did, nonetheless, organic food is higher in nutrients than its non-organic counterparts. And if you can obtain food produce from a biodynamic farm, it will have a much higher nutrient count again, as these farmers believe in maintaining the natural ecosystem of the soil and cultivating their crops as close to nature's way as possible. And of course, you could also grow your own.

Organic food produce, however, is quite expensive, and most of us are on a budget these days. So what can we do to help promote good health and less toxicity through food choices?

Every year, two new lists are produced by America's Environmental Working Group (EWG) and these lists are called the 'The Clean Fifteen' and 'The Dirty Dozen'. 'The Clean Fifteen' list is composed of the 15 non-organically grown fruits and vegetables that, when tested, had less chemical residue on them than any of the others. This makes them safer to consume than any of the others. 'The Dirty Dozen' list contains the twelve highest chemically-laden fruits and vegetables when tested against all the others, making these the least safe fruits and vegetables to eat. As such, it is advised not to eat any of the fruits and vegetables on 'The Dirty Dozen' list (below) unless they are organic. In conclusion, if you don't have very much money, then spend it on the organic versions of 'The Dirty Dozen', and don't worry too much about the others, as they have a lighter toxic load (just make sure to wash them all properly though, preferably in vinegar and water or bicarb and water).

Below is the UK version of these two essential lists. (2017)

Clean Fifteen

1. Sweetcorn
2. Avocados
3. Pineapple
4. Cabbage
5. Onions

6. Frozen sweet peas

7. Papayas

8. Asparagus

9. Mangos

10. Aubergine

11. Honeydew melon

12. Kiwi

13. Cantaloupe

14. Cauliflower

15. Grapefruit

Dirty Dozen

1. Strawberries

2. Spinach

3. Nectarines

4. Apples

5. Peaches

6. Pears

7. Cherries

8. Grapes

9. Celery

10. Tomatoes

11. Sweet bell peppers

12. Potatoes

Helpful Hints:

❀ It is advisable to soak all non-organic fruits and vegetables in a bicarb and water or vinegar solution to remove as much of the chemicals as possible before eating. Add 100 – 200ml of white or brown vinegar to a sink full of fresh (preferably filtered) water, add fruits and vegetables and let soak for at least 15 minutes, but preferably 1 hour. Remove, dry off and use.

❀ I have found that if you buy your produce directly from an organic farmer, it will work out much cheaper than buying the non-organic alternatives in your shops, so search out your local organic farmer.

❀ There are quite a few food co-ops around these days. These are groups of people that get together to buy in bulk, direct from the food source, which means the food is bought at a much lower price than what you would pay on your own. Have a search online for your local food co-op.

❀ Most countries in the world have their own versions of 'The Clean Fifteen' and 'The Dirty Dozen', and these change slightly from year to year, so it's always best to look up your local and most recent one, before you go off shopping.

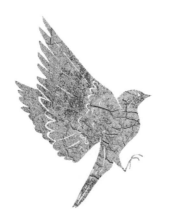

CHAPTER 11

HEALTHY RECIPES

*The first wealth is health – **Ralph Waldo Emerson***

This chapter has some ideas for menus that are easy, 'free-from' and healthy, that help stabilise blood sugar levels and hormones, and break cravings and addictions to food. These meals will minimise the amounts of toxins absorbed by your body, and they will support your body to eliminate the ones that are already on board.

Remember also to drink plenty of water, herbal teas and fermented drinks throughout your day to promote detoxification and balance blood sugars and hormones.

Note: I'm a vegetarian, and I eat no dairy, so where I have used a meat substitute, such as tofu or beans/pulses, feel free to use organic meat, fish or dairy instead.

BREAKFAST RECIPES

Brown Rice Pancakes

Makes 2 pancakes

Ingredients

75g cooked brown rice

1 egg white

250ml unsweetened almond milk

1 tbsp. ground hemp powder

1 tbsp. ground flax/linseed

1 tsp. cinnamon

coconut oil for frying

Directions

1. Put all the ingredients, apart from the oil, into a food processor and blend well.

2. Make mixture into two balls.

3. Add coconut oil to a frying pan and heat.

4. Add one of the balls to the pan and flatten to make a pancake shape, and cook for a few minutes until lightly browned. Flip and then do the same on the other side.

Amaranth Breakfast Cereal

Serves 4

Ingredients

500ml water (or almond milk)

180g amaranth seeds

1 tsp. cinnamon

1 tsp. chia seeds

sliced apple (optional)

berries, fresh or dried (optional)

dates (optional)

Directions

1. Put amaranth seeds in a pan of boiling water, turn down heat after two minutes and then allow to simmer for 20 minutes or until it gets thick.

2. Remove from heat and add cinnamon and chia seeds. Let sit a few minutes to allow chia seeds to expand. Serve hot.

Granola

Makes 10 portions

Ingredients

75g sunflower seeds

50g pumpkin seeds

50g flax/linseeds

50g chia seeds

90g shelled hazelnuts, roughly chopped

125g buckwheat flakes

125g rice flakes

125g millet flakes

1 tbsp. cinnamon

115g dried apple, roughly chopped (optional)

115g dried, stoned dates, roughly chopped (optional)

1 tbsp. honey (optional)

Directions

1. Soak seeds and hazelnuts for 3 hours or more. When ready to use, drain, rinse well and dry. Combine the mix with cinnamon and honey.
2. Place in a dehydrator for 14-16 hours or place in the bottom of a conventional oven at very low heat for an hour or until completely dried out.
3. Place mixture in a large bowl and allow to cool.
4. Combine the mixture thoroughly with other fruits you desire.
5. Store in an airtight container.

Note: You can use a combination of as many seeds and nuts as you wish and even add gluten-free oats.

Porridge

Serves 4

Ingredients

225g millet flakes or gluten-free oats

450ml dairy-free milk (I prefer almond milk)

salt (a pinch of ground sea salt)

a pinch nutmeg or cinnamon

Directions

1. Put millet/oats, milk and salt in a large saucepan. Bring to boil, then turn down heat. Stirring constantly, simmer for 5 minutes until creamy.

2. Place in a bowl and sprinkle with nutmeg or cinnamon.

Broccoli Hash

Serves 4

Ingredients

400g sweet potatoes

175g broccoli (cut into small florets)

2 tbsp. olive oil

1 onion (finely chopped)

1 large red pepper (diced)

½ tsp. dried chilli flakes

salt and pepper to taste

Directions

1. Place sweet potatoes in a pan of boiling water with a pinch of salt just for taste. Drain, once cooked.

2. Slightly steam the broccoli for 3 minutes.

3. In a large frying pan, heat oil over high heat. Add the onion and red pepper and fry for 2 minutes or until soft.

4. Add potatoes to frying pan and stir occasionally, for 6-8 minutes until soft.

5. Add the broccoli and chilli flakes to the frying pan and turn down heat. Fry until the mixture is lightly browned.

Oat and Ginger Granola

Serves 4

Ingredients

270g gluten-free oats

1 tbsp. chia seeds soaked for at least one hour

2 tbsp. gluten-free flour

1 tsp. cinnamon

1 tbsp. shredded coconut

40g pecans soaked for at least one hour and chopped

150g cashews soaked for at least one hour and chopped

80g walnuts soaked for at least one hour and chopped

¼ tsp. ground ginger

40g pumpkin seeds soaked for at least one hour

¼ tsp Himalayan salt

1-2 tbsp. coconut oil

100g dates chopped (optional)

Directions

1. Preheat oven to 325°F / 170°C / gas mark 3.

2. Put all the ingredients in a large bowl and mix well. Evenly spread the granola onto a baking sheet and bake, stirring occasionally, for about 30 minutes or until golden brown.

Sweet Potato and Courgette Hash Browns

Serves 4

Ingredients

1 medium sweet potato, grated

2 courgettes, grated

½ tsp. Himalayan salt

1 small onion finely sliced

1 tsp. coconut oil

freshly ground black pepper to taste

Directions

1. Mix the grated courgettes with the Himalayan salt and place in a colander. Place a dish underneath the colander and set aside for 10 minutes. The salt will draw the liquid from the courgettes. Squeeze the excess liquid from the courgettes until very dry, blot with a towel and place them in the mixing bowl with the grated sweet potato and onion. Mix well.

2. Taste and add more salt and freshly ground black pepper if desired, then make into balls.

3. Preheat a frying pan over medium heat and add the oil. Once the oil is hot, add the hash browns. Press them down into the pan using the back of a spatula. Cook for 3-6 minutes.

4. When the hash browns are slightly golden, flip them over and cook for another 3-6 minutes.

5. Remove from heat and serve immediately, or allow to cool down and freeze for next time. I like to make up big batches of these so I have them in the freezer when needed. I then reheat them in the oven.

Detox Smoothie

Serves 1

Ingredients

½ a large cucumber, chopped

2 large handfuls of kale

1 large handful of spinach

1 handful of fresh parsley

200ml of unsweetened raw coconut water

1 small handful of ice

¼ tbsp. of grated ginger

1 tsp of spirulina

1 tsp chia seeds

juice of one lemon

water

Directions

1. Place all the ingredients in a blender and top up with water.

2. Blend until smooth.

Immunity-Building Smoothie

Serves 1

Ingredients

¼ tbsp. of grated ginger

1 small cucumber chopped

2 large handfuls of spinach

1 handful of sprouted seeds

200ml of unsweetened raw coconut water

juice of ½ lemon

optional: 1 cup berries of your choice

water

Directions

1. Place all the ingredients in a blender and top up with water.

2. Blend until smooth.

Hormonal-Balancing Maca Smoothie

Serves 1

Ingredients

1 stalk of celery

½ a large cucumber

1 head of lettuce, chopped, with the core removed

1 tbsp of maca powder

½ tsp of organic matcha powder

1 scoop of raw vanilla powder (like Sunwarrior)

½ tsp cinnamon

1 tbp chia seeds

small handful of ice

200ml raw coconut milk

optional – 1 tsp cacao nibs

water

Directions

3. Place all the ingredients in a blender and top up with water.

4. Blend until smooth.

Protein Smoothie

Serves 1

Ingredients

1 banana, peeled and chopped

1 large handful of berries

5-7 large basil leaves

1 large handful of kale or spinach

1 tbsp. tahini or other nut or seed butter

2 tbsp. hemp seeds

1 tsp of chia seeds

1 tsp of flax/linseeds

water

Directions

1. Place all the ingredients in a blender and top up with water.

2. Blend until smooth.

Smoothie Bowl

Serves 1

Ingredients

1 small cucumber, chopped

2 handfuls of berries

1 large handful of kale

1 large banana, peeled and chopped

1 pear (or apple), chopped

juice of 1 orange

1 handful of fresh mint

2 tbsp chia seeds

water

Directions

1. Place all the ingredients in a blender and top up with water.

2. Blend until smooth.

3. Pour into a bowl and top with your favourite granola and goji berries

Green Smoothie

Serves 1

Ingredients

1 avocado

¼ large cucumber, chopped

1 stick celery, chopped

1 tbsp. chia seeds (soaked for at least one hour)

1 tbsp. ground flax and hemp seeds

500ml filtered water or coconut water

1 good handful spinach or leafy greens

1 scoop vanilla raw protein powder

Directions

4. Place all ingredients into your smoothie maker or blender and blitz until smooth.

5. Sometimes I add juiced down beetroot, berries or other vegetables and fruits to this mix.

6. I recommend you eat all smoothies with a spoon so that your saliva can mix with your food and start the digestive process working.

Note: You do not have to have breakfast foods for breakfast: bean, rice or quinoa salads are also a great way to start the day.

LUNCH RECIPES

Protein-Packed Broccoli Salad

Serves 4-6

Ingredients

1 head of broccoli, cut into small pieces

100g of walnuts, chopped into smaller pieces (maybe quarters)

1 large red onion, cut into thin slices

1-2 large handful(s) of pumpkin seeds

3-4 tbsp. of tahini

1 tbsp. of seaweed flakes

juice of a small lemon or lime

2 tbsp. maple syrup (or honey if you prefer)

¼ tsp. garlic power

2-3 tbsp. boiling water

Directions

1. Place all your vegetables, nuts and seeds in a large bowl and mix

2. In a separate, smaller bowl add all the other ingredients except for the hot water and mix

3. Then add the hot water to make the dressing thinner and slightly runny

4. Once you have your desired consistency, add the dressing to the vegetables etc. and mix well, so that everything gets covered in the dressing

5. Place in the fridge for 2-3 hours to marinate and so the broccoli softens slightly

Spinach, Pine Nut and Avocado Salad

Serves 4

Ingredients

60g small spinach leaves

16 cherry tomatoes

60g lamb's lettuce (or other soft lettuce or leaves of your choice)

30g pine nuts

1 tbsp. lime juice

1 tbsp. sesame seed oil

1 tsp. dried seaweed flakes

3 spring onions

1 large avocado

Directions

1. Put spinach leaves and lettuce in a bowl.
2. Cube the avocado flesh, halve the cherry tomatoes and slice the spring onion.
3. Toast the pine nuts in a medium oven or grill and add to the bowl.
4. Add lime juice, sesame seed oil and seaweed and mix well. Allow to sit for at least one hour before serving.

Spicy Tomato Soup

Serves 4

Ingredients

1 large onion

2 garlic cloves

1 tbsp. olive oil

1 large carrot

1 large courgette

1 medium sweet potato

600ml passata sauce

1 litre water or gluten-free vegetable stock

1-2 tsp. paprika

1 tsp. dried oregano

2 tbsp. chopped fresh basil

1 tbsp. chopped fresh coriander

1 tbsp. chopped fresh parsley

salt and freshly ground black pepper

¼-½ tsp chilli powder (optional)

Directions

1. Finely dice onion and then lightly fry in a pan with a little oil.
2. Crush the garlic cloves, take off the skin and add to onions.
3. Grate the carrot, courgette and sweet potato and add to the onions. Return to steaming the vegetables, stirring from time to time, until they begin to soften and brown.
4. Add the passata, water or stock, paprika, chilli powder and oregano to mixture in saucepan. Boil and then simmer for an extra 15 minutes or until vegetables are tender.
5. Add the fresh herbs and season to taste with salt and black pepper (optional). Simmer for 2 more minutes and serve.

Sprout and Mushroom Soup

Serves 4-6 (you can just add water the next day and it goes a long way)

Ingredients

300g of mushrooms, sliced

400g of brussels sprouts, remove outer leaves and cut in half

2 yellow onions, peeled and finely chopped

150g of uncooked brown rice

4 garlic cloves, peeled and finely chopped or minced

1 tsp of dried thyme

1 tsp of dried oregano

4 dried bay leaves (removed before serving)

1 tbsp. olive oil

1.5 litres of vegetable stock

1 tsp. miso paste (optional)

¼ tsp. of fresh ground pepper

Himalayan salt or sea salt to taste

Directions

1. Heat the oil in a large saucepan, add the onions and sprouts and cook until soft

2. Add garlic and mushrooms and cook until the mushrooms are soft

3. Add stock, rice, bay leaves and other herbs and leave to simmer for 45 minutes

4. Remove the bay leaves and season to taste and serve

5. To reheat the following day, add an additional ½ litre of stock before heating

Cream of Mushroom Soup

Serves 4

Ingredients

400g of mushrooms, sliced

2 yellow onions, peeled and finely chopped

1 tbsp. olive or nut oil

1 litre of vegetable stock

5 small garlic cloves, peeled and finely chopped or minced

200ml of vegan cream (check out the recipe for this later in this book)

200ml of nut milk

4 dried bay leaves (removed before blending)

¼ tsp. of fresh ground pepper

Himalayan salt or sea salt to taste

Directions

1. Heat the oil in a large saucepan, add the onions and cook until soft

2. Add garlic and mushrooms and cook until the mushrooms are soft

3. Add stock, bay leaves and pepper and leave to simmer for 45 minutes

4. Add cream and milk and cooked for a further 15 minutes

5. Season to taste and leave to cool

6. Once cooled, remove bay leaves and blend soup and return to saucepan and heat through again and serve

Optional: serve with a little freshly chopped parsley and a drizzle of vegan cream

Spicy Squash Soup

Serves 4

Ingredients

1 medium butternut squash (or pumpkin), peeled, de-seeded
and chopped into small cubes

3 yellow onions, peeled and finely chopped

1 tbsp. olive or nut oil

1 litre of vegetable stock

juice of half a lemon

5 small garlic cloves, peeled and finely chopped or minced

¼ tsp. of ground cayenne pepper

¼ tsp. ground paprika

4 dried bay leaves (removed before blending)

¼ tsp. of fresh ground pepper

Himalayan salt or sea salt to taste

Directions

1. Heat the oil in a large saucepan, add the onions and cook until
   soft
2. Add garlic, cayenne and paprika and cook for another 5 minutes
3. Add stock, bay leaves, lemon and pepper and leave to simmer
   for 45 minutes
4. Season to taste and leave to cool
5. Once cooled, blend soup and return to saucepan and heat
   through again and serve
6. Optionally, serve with a little vegan cream poured over the top
   and fresh parsley

Thai Tofu Cakes

Serves 8

Ingredients

300g firm tofu drained and crumbled down

1 lemon grass stalk, outer layer discarded, finely chopped

2 garlic cloves, chopped

1-inch piece fresh ginger, grated

2 shallots, finely chopped

2 fresh red chillies, deseeded and finely chopped

4 tbsp. chopped fresh coriander

90g gluten-free plain flour, plus extra for flouring

½ tsp. salt

2-3 tbsp. coconut oil, for frying

2 kaffir lime leaves, finely chopped (optional)

Directions

1. Combine the tofu with the lemon grass, garlic, ginger, lime leaves if using, shallots, chillies and coriander in a mixing bowl.

2. Stir in the flour and salt to make a coarse, sticky paste. Allow the mixture to firm up slightly by covering and chilling it in the refrigerator.

3. Flour your hands and form the mixture into small balls. Use your hands to flatten into rounds until you have 8 cakes.

4. Add oil to a large frying pan and place over medium heat. Cook the cakes for 4-6 minutes or until golden brown, turn and cook for the same amount of time on the other side.

5. Drain on paper towel and serve with salad, rice or quinoa.

Tortilla, Spanish Style

Serves 4

Ingredients

450g selection of peppers, onions, peas, sweet potatoes, courgettes and greens

1tbsp. olive oil

4 eggs

200ml dairy-free milk

2 tbsp. rice flour

1 large tomato

salt and freshly ground black pepper

Directions

1. Cut vegetables into small cubes.
2. Put them in a saucepan with olive oil and allow to slightly steam until they become soft and brown.
3. Combine eggs, milk and rice flour and beat into a batter, then season with salt and black pepper.
4. Put the vegetables in a greased flan dish or oven-proof bowl and pour the egg mixture over the top.
5. Carefully slice the tomato and put the slices on the top of the tortilla.
6. In a preheated oven 325°F/170°C /gas mark 3, bake for approximately 30 minutes or until the tortilla begins brown. Cut into wedges and serve with a salad garnish.

Oriental Rice Salad

Serves 4

Ingredients

125g brown rice

2 tbsp. sesame oil

2 tbsp. lime juice

1 tsp. grated fresh ginger

30g flaked almonds (soaked for at least one hour and patted down)

30g sunflower seeds (soaked for at least one hour and patted down)

60g sesame seeds (soaked for at least one hour and patted down)

freshly ground black pepper

Directions

1. Brown rice should be cooked until tender in lots of water. Drain excess water.
2. Add lime juice, grated ginger, sesame oil to the warm rice and mix. Then allow rice to cool.
3. The almonds, sunflower seeds and sesame seeds should be placed in a medium oven for around 20 minutes, stirring part way through.
4. Combine the nuts and seeds with lots of black pepper with the rice immediately before serving.

Scrambled Tofu or Vegetable Tofu Scramble

Serves 4

Ingredients

120ml and 1 tbsp. coconut oil, divided

1 to 2 cloves garlic, minced

1 tsp. sesame seed oil

¼ tsp. dried flaked seaweed

¼ tsp. sea salt

1 pack of firm tofu, drained

1 onion, chopped

¼ head of broccoli, chopped

1 pepper, deseeded and chopped

2 to 4 tbsp. torn fresh basil

½ tsp. fresh cracked pepper

¼ tsp. sea salt (optional)

4 mushrooms, chopped (optional)

¼ tsp. chilli flakes (optional)

Directions

1. Combine 120ml oil, garlic, sesame seed oil, seaweed, sea salt (and chilli flakes if adding these) in casserole dish.
2. Mix well, then crumble the drained tofu into the mixture and put aside to marinate.
3. Over medium heat, heat a large pan and add the tablespoon of coconut oil. Sauté onion and peppers until soft, then add the remaining vegetables and cook until lightly brown.
4. Drain the marinated tofu, add it to the pan and warm through.
5. Put in the basil and stir, then season with salt and pepper to taste. Heat thoroughly and serve immediately.
6. You can add brown rice or quinoa to this for a heartier meal.

Lentil and Coconut Soup

Serves 4

Ingredients

2 large onions

600ml gluten-free vegetable stock

1 clove garlic

90g creamed coconut

2 tsp. grated fresh ginger

850ml water

1 tbsp. olive oil

1 tbsp. tomato paste, optional

1 heaped tsp. ground coriander

1 tsp. ground cardamom

1 tsp. ground cinnamon

¼ tsp. ground cloves

175g red split lentils

fresh parsley, to garnish

salt and freshly ground black pepper

Directions

1. Dice onions, crush garlic and place them in saucepan along with the olive oil and ginger. Lightly steam them until the onions are soft and brown.

2. Combine the coriander, cardamom, cinnamon and cloves and place them in the pan, then slightly steam the mix for a few minutes.

3. Place the split lentils and stock in pan, simmer for 20-25 minutes or until lentils are soft.

4. Put the soup in a food processor and blend until silky smooth. If you do not have a food processor, you can sieve to purée the mixture.

5. Boil 300ml of the water, add the creamed coconut and stir until mixed well.

6. Add the balance of water, tomato paste, and salt and black pepper to taste.

7. Heat thoroughly, garnish with chopped parsley and serve.

Quinoa and Edamame Salad

Serves 4

Ingredients

130g quinoa

1 red pepper, finely diced

200g shelled edamame

40g chopped walnuts, preferably toasted

1 tbsp. lemon zest

2 tbsp. lemon juice

2 tbsp. olive oil

500ml yeast-free vegetable stock

2 tbsp. chopped fresh tarragon or 2 tsp. dried

½ tsp. Himalayan salt or sea salt

Directions

1. Toast quinoa in a dry pan over a medium heat until it becomes to crackle. Do not allow it to burn. Rinse thoroughly with water.

2. Use the same pan to light toast the walnuts for no more than 4 minutes and set aside.

3. Bring your stock to boil in a large saucepan and add the. Reduce to a simmer, cover and cook for 8 minutes.

4. Add edamame, cover and continue to cook until everything is tender, about 8 minutes more. Drain any remaining water.

5. Add all remaining ingredients apart from the pepper and walnuts to a bowl and whisk well.

6. Add the pepper and the quinoa mixture to the bowl and mix well.

7. Serve and top with walnuts.

Falafel Patties

Makes 8

Ingredients

300g pre-soaked/sprouted and cooked chickpeas (or well-rinsed canned)

50g gram flour

6 cloves garlic, minced

1 red onion finely chopped

1 handful fresh parsley, chopped

1 tbsp. cumin

¼ tsp. cayenne pepper or chilli powder

1 tsp. coriander

¼ tsp. Himalayan salt

½ tsp. fresh cracked pepper

coconut oil for frying

Directions

1. Put all the ingredients except the oil for frying in a food processor and blend for a minute or until smooth. Add small amount of water to the mixture if it is too thick.
2. Put mixture in medium-size bowl and place in fridge overnight.
3. Remove mixture from refrigerator. Make 2-inch diameter patties and place on a plate. Add water if patties crumble: this will ensure that they hold firmly together.
4. Heat approximately 2 tbsp. of oil in a pan over medium heat. When hot, add patties and cook for 3-4 minutes or until crispy on either side.
5. If more oil is needed you can add as you go along. Place patties on paper towels to drain.

Quinoa Falafel

Serves 4-5

Ingredients

250g cooked quinoa

2 eggs, lightly beaten

30g almond flour

3 tbsp. gram flour (or any other free-from flour)

1 large onion, finely chopped

4 tbsp. fresh parsley, chopped

1 clove garlic, finely chopped

½ tsp. ground cumin

½ tsp. ground coriander

1 tsp. Himalayan salt or sea salt

¼ tsp pepper

2 tbsp. olive oil

Directions

1. Add all ingredients to a large bowl and mix well.
2. Make 24 balls out of the mixture, which are all roughly the same size.
3. Add the oil to a frying pan and heat. Add half the balls and fry until golden, stirring often.
4. Remove and drain on kitchen paper whilst cooking the other half and then drain in the same way.
5. Serve with a salad, fresh parsley and a dip of your choice.

Fritters

Serves 4

Ingredients

125g gluten-free self-raising flour

1 egg (beaten)

175ml unsweetened dairy-free milk

140g spring onions, thinly sliced

400g canned chickpeas, well rinsed and drained

4 tbsp. chopped coriander or parsley

100 – 150ml of coconut oil (enough for ½ cm depth at the bottom of the pan)

salt and pepper

Directions

1. Pour flour into a sieve and sift into a bowl, then combine with egg and milk. Stir, then whisk gently for a smooth batter.
2. Add the other ingredients except the oil to the batter mix, add salt and pepper.
3. In a large pan, heat the oil, and pour in 1 tbsp. of batter at a time to make small fritters.
4. Allow fritters to fry for 5 minutes, turning so that both sides are lightly browned.
5. Serve fritters with salad and dips.

Vegan Fish Cakes

Makes 8 fish cakes

Ingredients

2 medium sweet potatoes, peeled

1 can of butter beans, rinsed and drained

1 large courgette grated

130g gluten-free flour

25ml of sesame seed oil

3 tsp. of seaweed flakes

1 tsp. hot paprika

1 tsp. Himalayan salt or sea salt

½ tsp. pepper

coconut oil for frying

Directions

1. Cut the potatoes into small chunks, place in a saucepan and boil until tender.
2. Rinse with cold water and put in a food processor with the beans, sesame seed oil, seaweed, paprika, salt and pepper and blend until smooth and set aside.
3. Squeeze out any excess water from the courgettes.
4. Add the courgette and the potato mix to a large bowl and add half the gluten-free flour and mix well.
5. Put the remaining flour on a large plate and heat the oil in a large flat frying pan.
6. Split the mixture into eight equal pieces and roll each piece into a ball.
7. Roll each ball in the flour on the plate, covering fully and then flatten into patty shapes and then fry for 3 to 4 minutes on each side until golden.

Cauliflower Wraps

Makes 2 wraps

Ingredients

½ head cauliflower, cut into small pieces

2 eggs

1 garlic clove, minced

½ tsp. dried basil or a small handful of chopped fresh basil

¼ tsp. Himalayan or sea salt

Directions

1. Preheat your oven to 350°F/180°C/gas mark 6.
2. Line a baking tray with greaseproof paper.
3. Blend the cauliflower in a food processor until it's crumbled down.
4. Place the cauliflower in a pan of boiling water with a lid on it and boil for 10 minutes.
5. Drain the cauliflower and then squeeze the excess water from the
6. cauliflower through a tea-towel.
7. Place the cauliflower and all the remaining ingredients in a large bowl and stir well.
8. Separate the ingredients into two halves and make flat round wrap shapes out of each on the greaseproof paper.
9. Bake for 15 to 20 minutes (making sure they don't harden and are still able to bend like a wrap.
10. Allow to dry on a wire rack.
11. Fill with salad, hummus and/or avocado and/or a protein of your choice.

Roasted Vegetables

Serves 2

Ingredients

350g fresh vegetables, such as broccoli, cauliflower, radish, carrots, celery and courgette

1 large chard leaf, sliced into ribbons

2 tbsp. crushed almonds

1 clove garlic, thinly sliced

½ tsp. red pepper flakes

½ tsp. ground turmeric powder

¼ tsp. ground cayenne powder

¼ tsp. ground curry powder

1 tsp. Himalayan salt or sea salt

1 tbsp. olive oil for drizzling

2 tbsp. sesame seed oil

Directions

1. Preheat your oven to 350°F/180°C/gas mark 6.
2. Place all the vegetables on a baking tray, drizzle with oil and sprinkle with the salt, turmeric, cayenne and curry powder.
3. Roast vegetables for 15 minutes, turning once half way through cooking.
4. Add the roasted vegetables and all other ingredients into a large bowl and mix well.
5. Serve as is, or with some quinoa.

DINNER RECIPES
Spicy Bean & Quinoa Salad

Serves 4

Ingredients

100g quinoa (I like red in this meal, but any colour works)

1 red pepper, chopped

1 red or white onion, chopped

1 can of cooked beans of your choice, rinsed well, (I like a mixed can of beans)

1 garlic clove, finely chopped

1 handful of parsley, chopped

1 handful of coriander, chopped

½ tsp. cayenne pepper, ground

½ tsp. paprika, ground

¼ tsp. ginger, ground

2 tbsp. olive oil (or sesame seed oil works really well too)

juice of one lime

salt and pepper to taste

Directions

1. Cook quinoa as per directions on the package (you can also add a stock cube whilst cooking for a greater depth of flavour).

2. Add oil and cayenne and paprika to a pan and slightly fry the onion and peppers until soft, then add the garlic and fry for another couple of minutes (making sure not to burn).

3. Place quinoa, onion and pepper mix and beans to a large bowl and mix well.

4. Add all the remaining ingredients (this works really well if still hot as it softens everything else.

5. Mix and serve warm or cold.

Polenta Pizza

Serves 4

Ingredients for the polenta pizza crust

110g polenta meal

1 tsp. dried basil

½ tsp. dried oregano

½ tsp. dried parsley

700ml of yeast-free stock

1 tsp. Himalayan or sea salt

2 tbsp. olive oil

For the topping

1 pepper, thinly sliced

1 onion, thinly sliced

2 large tomatoes, thinly sliced

1 bunch kale, finely chopped

3 tbsp. extra virgin olive oil

3 tbsp. sesame seed oil

For the walnut pesto

2 garlic cloves, peeled

60g walnuts, toasted

2 large handfuls of fresh basil

1 large handful of fresh spinach

50ml olive oil, plus more if needed

Himalayan or sea salt and black pepper to taste

Directions

1. Preheat the oven to 350°F/180°C/gas mark 6 and grease two
    11-inch flan tins.

2. Bring the stock to the boil in a large saucepan and immediately reduce to a simmer and add the crust herbs, salt, pepper, oil and polenta.

3. Make sure to whisk the ingredients continuously for at least 5 minutes and until smooth.

4. Pour half the mixture into one tin and half into the other one and allow to cool on the side before placing in the refrigerator for 30 minutes.

5. Remove polenta from refrigerator and place on some greaseproof paper on two baking trays and bake for 30 minutes.

6. Add all the pesto ingredients to a food processor and blend for 5 minutes and then spread evenly over the pizza bases.

7. Mix all topping ingredients really well in a large bowl, massaging all the oil and other ingredients well into the vegetables. Lay topping out on the two pizza bases equally.

8. Bake pizzas for a further 15 minutes and serve immediately.

9. You may wish to add your choice of protein to this pizza before baking the second time.

Chickpea Curry

Serves 4

Ingredients

2 cans of chickpeas

1 can of chopped tomatoes

4 large handful of chopped spinach

1 onion, finely chopped

½ tsp. ground ginger powder

½ tsp. ground garlic powder

½ tsp. ground chilli powder

½ tsp. ground turmeric powder

½ tsp. ground garam masala powder

½ tsp. Himalayan or sea salt

coconut or olive oil for frying

Directions

1. Rinse the chickpeas and set aside.
2. Add the oil to a fry pan and fry the onion until golden.
3. Add garlic, ginger, chilli powder, salt, turmeric and garam masala and stir well.
4. Add the tomatoes and spinach and stir again.
5. Add the chickpeas and simmer for 20 minutes.
6. Serve with brown rice or quinoa.

Pasta Ratatouille

Serves 4-5

Ingredients

1 small aubergine, chopped into small squares

1 courgette, chopped into small squares

1 sweet potato, chopped into small squares

2 small red onions, peeled and cut into wedges

2 to 4 garlic cloves, peeled and left whole

1-2 tbsp. olive oil

200g tomatoes (if fresh then chop into small pieces)

175g free-from pasta

handful of fresh basil, chopped

Directions

1. Preheat the oven to 350°F/180°C/gas mark 6.
2. Place all the chopped vegetables and garlic in a roasting tin, drizzle oil over vegetables and mix well.
3. Roast for 45 minutes, stirring half way through
4. Cook the pasta, drain and put back into pan.
5. Add the roasted vegetables, basil and tomatoes to pan and cook through, stirring well.

Three Bean Chilli

Serves 4

Ingredients

60g aduki beans

60g red kidney beans

60g whole red lentils

1 large onion

1 sweet green pepper

1 large carrot

1 green chilli

1 clove garlic

2 tsp. coconut oil

600ml passata sauce

1 bay leaf

1 tsp. dried basil

1 tsp. dried oregano

¼-½ tsp. chilli powder

salt and freshly ground black pepper

Directions

1. Prepare lentils by soaking them in lots of water overnight. Before cooking, rinse and place in pot with enough water to cover them. Boil and simmer until beans are tender.

2. Cut vegetables very finely. Remove seeds from chilli and dice, crush garlic cloves.

3. In a saucepan with coconut oil, place the vegetables, chilli and garlic, then steam them slightly or until they are soft.

4. Add the passata, herbs, spices, the beans and their cooking liquid, plus adequate water, if necessary, to make a runny sauce.

5. Boil and simmer until all the vegetables and beans are tender and the sauce is thick. Simmer until the lentils and beans start to break down, this will allow them to form a part of the sauce.

6. Season with salt and black pepper and serve.

Seaweed and Tofu Stir-Fry

Serves 2

Ingredients

2 strips of dried kombu kelp

1 carrot (and/or baby sweetcorn)

1 white onion

¼ tsp. chilli pepper

4 tbsp. sesame oil

half a pack of firm tofu, drained and sliced into cubes

Directions

1. Add the kombu to some water and soak for at least one hour.
2. Fry tofu in a pan with half the sesame seed oil, making sure to turn regularly until the tofu is browned on all sides. Set aside.
3. Cut kombu into strips, then do the same with the carrot and baby sweetcorn (if using these).
4. Slice the onion thinly.
5. Pour the remaining oil into a wok and stir-fry all the other ingredients apart from the tofu and kombu. Add the remaining ingredients when everything else is cooked through.
6. Serve immediately, either on its own or with quinoa.

Deconstructed Vegan Moussaka

Serves 4 – 6

Ingredients

2 medium aubergines, chopped into small chunks

2 small courgettes, chopped into small chunks

5 large potatoes, peeled and cut into small chunks

1 large onion, peeled and chopped

2 cans of chopped tomatoes

500 – 700ml of yeast-free vegetable stock

200g of red split pea lentils

1 jar (and oil) of sundried tomatoes, sliced

6 cloves garlic, peeled

2-3 bay leaves

2 cinnamon sticks

5 tbs. dried oregano

½-1 tsp. nutmeg or mustard powder

50ml almond milk (or dairy-free milk)

60ml of olive oil

½-1 tsp. of fresh ground pepper

Directions

1. Place the aubergine and courgette into a bowl, sprinkle with salt, mix well and set aside for at least 30 minutes (stir occasionally).
2. Add the olive oil to a large frying pan.
3. Add the onions, aubergine and courgette to cook until soft.
4. Add tomatoes, lentils, stock (just 500ml to start with), cinnamon, bay leaves, sundried tomatoes and their oil and oregano and stir well and bring to the boil and then reduce to simmer for 40 – 60 minutes, making sure everything is tender. You may need to add the rest of the stock if it gets a bit dry.

5. Stir regularly or the lentils will stick to the bottom

6. After about 20 minutes, cook potatoes for roughly 20 minutes until soft. Drain, add almond milk and nutmeg or mustard and mash well.

7. Remove lentil mix from the heat season with salt and pepper if desired, remove the cinnamon sticks and bay leaves and serve.

8. Place mashed potatoes on top and serve as is, or place under the grill until golden.

Indian-Style Roasted Vegetables with Pilau Rice and Dahl

Serves 4

Ingredients for the Dahl

175g red split lentils

1tsp. cumin seeds

½ tsp. turmeric

½ tsp. ground coriander

½ tsp. grated fresh ginger

1 garlic clove, crushed

¼ tsp. chilli powder

850ml water

salt and freshly ground black pepper

Roasted Vegetables Ingredients

2 medium carrots

2 red peppers

8 small onions

1 medium aubergine

3 medium courgettes

2 tsp. cumin seeds

2-3-inch piece fresh ginger

2-3 garlic cloves

1 tsp. ground coriander

½ tsp. chilli powder

¼ tsp. ground cardamom

¼ tsp. garam masala

3 tbsp. coconut oil

salt and freshly ground black pepper

Pilau Rice Ingredients

200g brown basmati rice

60g wild rice

1 heaped tsp. turmeric

60g raisins (optional)

Directions

1. Put all the dahl ingredients in a saucepan. Boil and simmer for 1 -1½ hours or until the dahl becomes smooth and thick. Ensure to stir occasionally to prevent lumping.

2. Crush the garlic cloves and grate the ginger finely. Using the back of a metal spoon, press the ginger and garlic through a sieve or use a juicer until you have approximately 1½ teaspoons of juice. Put this in a large bowl.

3. Combine chilli powder, cardamom, garam masala, coconut oil and coriander and whisk until silky smooth. Season to taste.

4. Cut onions into halves, sweet peppers into 8 pieces, courgettes and the aubergine into 1 cm / ½ inch slices.

5. Put the vegetables and coconut oil mixture in a bowl and toss until coated.

6. Put the vegetables on baking trays and sprinkle the cumin seeds on them.

7. Preheat oven at 400°F/200°C/gas mark 6 and bake for 30 minutes or until the vegetables are cooked and brown. Stir during cooking.

8. While vegetables are roasting, prepare the rice. Wash rice and put in a pan with 1.2 litres boiling water and add turmeric. Simmer for 20 minutes and add the raisins 1-2 minutes before end of cooking.

9. Sieve to remove excess liquid. Serve roasted vegetables with pilau rice; serve the dahl in a separate bowl.

Leek and Lentil Terrine

Serves 4

Ingredients for Lentil Mixture

225g split red lentils

750ml water

1 tsp. garam masala

½ tsp. paprika

½ tsp. turmeric

1 tsp. grated fresh ginger

1 egg

salt and freshly ground black pepper

Ingredients for Leek Mixture

1 egg

275g leeks, mainly white stems

175g fennel and/or celery

1 tsp. olive oil

60ml water

60g cashew nuts

90ml dairy-free milk

1tsp. ground fennel seeds

salt and freshly ground black pepper

Directions

1. Make the leek mixture by filling a saucepan with water. Add the lentils, garam masala, paprika, turmeric and grated ginger. Cook for 20 minutes or until lentils are soft. Allow to cool.

2. Slice the leeks and fennel finely, add these to a saucepan with olive oil. Slightly steam the vegetables until they are tender. Add water and simmer for 2-3 minutes or until vegetables are soft.

3. Grind the cashew nuts in a food processor. Add the milk,

fennel seeds, the egg and half of the cooked vegetables and process until smooth. Add this to the pan and combine with the remaining vegetables. Season to taste with salt and black pepper.

4. Make the lentil layer by placing the lentils, ginger and the egg in the food processor and process until smooth. Season to taste with salt and black pepper.

5. Lay half of the lentil mixture in a greased and lined loaf tin. Place leek mixture on top of the lentils to form another layer. Complete by adding another layer of lentils.

6. Bake, uncovered, in a preheated oven, 200°C/400°F/gas mark 6 for 45-55 minutes or until the top begins to brown and the loaf is set.

7. Let the terrine sit for 10 minutes before placing it on a serving dish. To serve, cut into slices and serve with vegetables or salad.

Vegetable and Ginger Casserole with Herb Dumplings

Serves 4

Ingredients

1.1 kg selection of swede, parsnips, carrots, onions, leeks, broccoli, courgettes, celery, peppers, pumpkin, celeriac

1-inch piece fresh ginger

400g tomatoes chopped

100g red split pea lentils

850ml water

1 tsp. paprika

1 tsp. fennel seeds

½ tsp. dried thyme

1 tsp. celery seeds

1 tbsp. chopped fresh coriander

1 tbsp. chopped fresh parsley

salt and freshly ground black pepper

For the dumplings

175g well-cooked brown rice

4 tsp. olive oil

125-180ml water

90g rice flour

2 tsp. baking powder

¼ tsp. dried thyme

salt and freshly ground black pepper

Directions

1. Cut the vegetables into large chunks of the same size and thinly slice the ginger.

2. In a casserole dish, put the tomatoes, lentils, water, spices, herbs, salt and black pepper, vegetables and ginger and mix well.

3. Cook in a preheated oven, 200°C/400°F/gas mark 6, for 1¼ hours.

4. In the meantime, prepare the dumplings. Place rice, oil and 125ml of water in a food processor and process until smooth.

5. Combine rice flour, baking powder, thyme, salt and black pepper. Add rice flour to the processor and process again, adding remaining 125ml water to make a soft dough. The amount of water will depend on how well cooked the rice is.

6. Make 12 dumplings from the mixture and roll them in a small amount of rice flour.

7. Add the dumplings to the top of the vegetable mix in the casserole dish. Put in the oven and cook for a further 15-20 minutes.

Lentil and Vegetable Curry (with optional egg)

Serves 4

Ingredients

200g split red lentils or puy lentils

1 litre water

780g selection of leeks, onions, celery, carrots, courgettes, sweet peppers, baby sweetcorn, okra

2 garlic cloves

1-inch piece fresh ginger

1 tbsp. coconut oil

1 tsp. ground cumin

1 tsp. ground coriander

½ tsp. garam masala

½ tsp. turmeric

¼ tsp. cayenne pepper or chilli powder

¼ tsp. ground cardamom

salt and freshly ground black pepper

4 eggs not quite hard-boiled, shelled and sliced into four (optional)

Directions

1. Cook lentils for approximately 1 hour in water or until they are soft, then purée them.
2. Grate ginger, crush garlic cloves, then cut the vegetables into same size chunks.
3. Put the vegetables in saucepan with the oil, slightly steam for a few minutes, then add garlic and ginger. Steam longer until garlic and ginger are soft.
4. Add the spices and cook for another 2 minutes.

5. Add lentil purée and simmer for 15 minutes. Add water if it becomes a little dry. Add eggs at this stage and warm through.

6. Salt and black pepper can be added for taste. Serve with rice or quinoa.

Black Bean Burgers

Makes 4 burgers

Ingredients

300g dried black beans, soaked, drained and cooked

2 tsp. dried parsley

3 tbsp. finely chopped onions

1 carrot, grated

1 tsp. chia seeds soaked in water for an hour

½ tsp. cumin

1 tsp. chilli powder

1 tsp. garlic, minced

40g gluten-free flour

2 tbsp. coconut oil

1 tsp. Himalayan salt

Directions

1. Put the beans in a food processor and blend, but not until smooth: mixture should be lumpy.
2. Add the other ingredients, except flour and coconut oil, to the mixture and blend until smooth. Pour into a bowl.
3. Add flour and form the mixture into burger-size patties. Place burgers onto a plate.
4. Heat coconut oil in a pan over medium heat. Cook burgers in pan for 4 minutes, turn and cook on the other side for a further 4 minutes. Watch them carefully, as they can burn easily.
5. Serve with salad.

Carrot, Parsnip and Cashew Nut Roast

Serves 4

Ingredients

450g carrots

175g parsnips

60g celery

1 large onion diced

90g quinoa

125g cashew nuts (soaked for at least 2 hours)

1 tsp. dried thyme

1 tsp. dried sage

1 tbsp. fresh parsley, chopped

1 clove garlic, diced

1 tbsp. olive oil

salt and freshly ground black pepper

Directions

1. Put carrots in a pan of boiling water and steam until soft, then transfer to a food processor and blend. Set aside.
2. Boil the quinoa as per the packet instructions, turn the heat off. Cover and leave to absorb the water for about half an hour and then drain.
3. Place cashews in a medium oven for 30 minutes, to dry out. Do not brown too much.
4. Place onions, garlic and celery in a saucepan with the olive oil, and sweat for 3 minutes.
5. Grate the parsnips and add to the pan. Cook over a medium heat, stirring occasionally, until light brown.
6. Combine all the ingredients with the carrots and mix well. Season with salt and black pepper.

7. Place in a greased loaf tin, cover with foil and bake in a preheated oven at 180°C/350°F/gas mark 4 for approximately 40 minutes.

8. Serve with salad or vegetables.

Protein-Packed Baked Sweet Potatoes

Serves 4

Ingredients

4 sweet potatoes

1 small onion, thinly sliced

1 garlic clove, minced

1 can of white beans, cooked, drained and rinsed

1 large bunch of kale, sliced thinly

1 large handful of parsley

¼ tsp. red pepper flakes

2 tbsp. olive oil

Himalayan or sea salt and pepper to taste

Directions

1. Preheat the oven to 350°F/180°C/gas mark 6.
2. Prick the sweet potatoes with a fork and place them on a baking tray and bake for about an hour.
3. About 15 minutes before the sweet potatoes will be ready, start to prepare the filling.
4. In a large saucepan heat the oil and cook the onions until soft but not brown.
5. Add the garlic, parsley and pepper flakes and stir well.
6. Now add the beans and cook for a few minutes longer, then add the kale and salt and pepper and cook for a further 5-7 minutes, stirring occasionally.
7. Take the potatoes out of the oven and slice them open, add the bean mixture into them and serve immediately.

Spicy Egg and Vegetable Fried Rice

Serves 2

Ingredients

150g cooked brown rice

1 yellow pepper

2 red onions (one roughly chopped and one thinly sliced)

2 carrots, sliced into ribbons

4 spring onions, cut lengthwise

3 eggs

2 red chillies

3 garlic cloves

4 tbsp. sesame seed oil

handful of parsley

Himalayan or sea salt to taste

Directions

1. Scramble the eggs in wok or frying pan and then remove the eggs and set aside.
2. Place the roughly chopped onion, half the chilli, the garlic and sesame seed oil in a food processor and blend until smooth.
3. Add the above mixture to the wok or frying pan and heat through.
4. Add the thinly-sliced onion, the rest of the chilli, yellow pepper and carrot to the wok and lightly stir-fry for a couple of minutes.
5. Now add the rice, stir well and cook for another couple of minutes.
6. Now add the eggs back in, the spring onion, parsley and salt and pepper to taste.
7. Serve immediately.

Vegetarian Haggis

Serves 4-5

Ingredients

1 white onion, finely chopped

2 cloves garlic, finely sliced

30ml olive oil

½ tin of red kidney beans, well cooked and rinsed

pinch of cayenne pepper or chilli powder

½ tsp. ground cinnamon

½ tsp. allspice, ground

pinch of nutmeg

3 carrots, grated

75g red lentils

juice of 1 lemon

500ml gluten-free vegetable stock

small bunch rosemary, strip the leaves and chop them finely

small bunch thyme, leaves stripped

50g gluten-free oatmeal or oat bran

75g white mushrooms, roughly chopped (optional)

Directions

1. In a medium-sized casserole, sweat the onions and garlic in the oil until soft.

2. Add the mushrooms (if using) and sauté until light brown.

3. Add the spices and continue cooking for a few minutes. Then add carrots, lentils and pour the stock into the pan, just covering the ingredients. Simmer, covered, until the lentils are soft.

4. Mash the beans roughly with a fork, then add them and the oatmeal to the pan. Add a little more stock if you think it's needed. The oatmeal should absorb the last of the stock: if it doesn't, then cook for a little longer. Season to taste.

5. Spoon out the haggis and serve with tatties (potatoes – sweet potatoes work just as well as white potatoes here) and neeps (turnips) and/or gluten-free oat cakes.

SNACK RECIPES

Vegetable Tempura

Serves 4

Ingredients for the Ginger Tofu Dip

250g soft silken tofu, drained

¾-inch piece ginger, chopped

1 small shallot, chopped

1 garlic clove, crushed

1 tbsp. sesame seed oil

2 tsp. rice vinegar

Batter ingredients

150g gluten-free plain flour

1 egg

200ml iced water

Nut oil, for deep-frying

500g of a selection of asparagus, baby carrots, baby corn, broccoli florets or mushrooms

salt and pepper

Directions

1. For the dip, put all the ingredients in a food processor, process until smooth and set aside.

2. For the batter, beat together the flour, egg, water, salt and pepper: it should be smooth.

3. Heat oil in a deep pan.

4. Dip the vegetables quickly into the batter, then deep-fry in batches for 1-2 minutes until they are crisp. Drain, and serve with dip whilst hot.

Faith Canter

Cauliflower Crackers

Makes 36

Ingredients

30g cauliflower, roughly chopped

50ml sesame seeds

70g flax/linseeds, ground

2 tbsp. chia seeds

100g sesame seeds for topping

1 tsp. Himalayan or sea salt

75ml cup water

3 tbsp. coconut oil, melted

Directions

1. Blend the cauliflower in a food processor until it is well crumbled.

2. Now add all the other ingredients and pulse for a bit longer until it forms a dough. Chill for 4 hours.

3. Preheat the oven to 350°F/180°C/gas mark 6 and place some greaseproof paper on a baking tray.

4. Make 36 small balls from the dough and roll the balls in the sesame seeds.

5. Place the balls on the greaseproof paper and flatten out to make cracker shapes.

6. Bake for 30 minutes and then turn crackers over and bake for another 30 minutes.

7. Allow to cool on a wire rack.

8. Serve with pâté, hummus or avocado.

Spiced Potato Wedges with Garlic Mayonnaise Dip

Serves 4

Ingredients

4 medium sweet potatoes

1 tbsp. lemon juice

2 tbsp. olive oil

¼ tsp. chilli powder

salt and freshly ground black pepper

chopped fresh herbs, to garnish

garlic mayonnaise (see Side Dishes recipes)

Directions

1. Cut the potatoes in half lengthways, and then cut each half into four wedges lengthways.

2. In a large bowl, mix together lemon juice, olive oil and chilli powder and season with salt and pepper.

3. Toss the potato wedges in the oil mixture until well coated.

4. Put the potatoes on a large baking tray and bake in a preheated oven 200°C/400°F/gas mark 6 for approximately 40-50 minutes or until brown and crisp on the outside, but soft on the inside.

5. Serve with fresh herbs and garlic mayo dip.

Oven-Roasted Kale Chips

Serves 4

Ingredients

1 large bunch of kale

40g coconut oil, melted

2 tbsp. sesame seed oil

½ tsp. garlic powder

½ tsp. red chilli flakes

1 tsp. Himalayan or sea salt

ground black pepper to taste

Directions

1. Preheat oven to 350°F/180°C/gas mark 6.
2. Rinse kale, and dry out completely.
3. Remove any woody stems from your kale and place the rest of the kale in a large bowl.
4. Place rest of the ingredients in the bowl with the kale and massage into the kale well.
5. Put the kale mixture on a baking tray and cook for 5 minutes and then stir well and return to oven for a further 5 minutes.
6. Serve as it is as a snack, or on the side of a salad.

Nori Vegetable Rolls

Makes 8 rolls

Ingredients

300g sunflower seeds (soaked at least 4 hours)

1 tbsp. dried seaweed

3 tsp. minced garlic

2 spring onions, chopped

180g spinach, chopped

8 sheets raw nori (untoasted)

2 carrots, thinly sliced lengthways

1 large cucumber or courgette, thinly sliced lengthways

1 large avocado, thinly sliced lengthways

50ml lemon or lime juice (optional)

Directions

1. Put first five ingredients into a food processor and process until smooth.
2. Place on each nori sheet a layer of spinach leaves, sunflower mix and then slices of carrot, cucumber and avocado along the edge closest to you.
3. Tightly roll the nori sheet into a sausage shape and seal the edge with a little warm water.
4. Slice into small discs.
5. Serve with salad and dips.

SIDE DISHES RECIPES

Eggless Egg Salad

Serves 2-3

Ingredients

3 celery stalks, finely chopped

1 red pepper, finely chopped

½ small white onion, finely chopped (optional)

350g cashews

175 ml water

15 ml lemon juice

1 tbsp. turmeric

1 clove garlic

1 tsp. Himalayan or sea salt

paprika, to garnish/taste

Directions

1. Add all ingredients except the celery and the pepper to a food processor and blend until smooth.

2. Put the celery, pepper and onion (if you are using one) into a large bowl and pour in the cashew mixture from your food processor and mix well.

3. Serve with salad, wraps or on crackers with a sprinkling of paprika.

Tabbouleh

Serves 4

Ingredients

175g quinoa (soaked overnight)

600ml water

10 cherry tomatoes, halved

half a large cucumber, diced

3 spring onions, sliced

juice of ½ lemon

2 tbsp. extra virgin olive oil

4 tbsp. chopped fresh mint

4 tbsp. chopped fresh coriander

4 tbsp. chopped fresh parsley

salt and pepper

Directions

1. Put quinoa in a saucepan and cover with water. Bring to the boil, then take off the heat and drain.
2. Leave the quinoa to cool for a few minutes before combining it with the remaining ingredients in a salad bowl.
3. Season to taste.

Aubergine and Sun-Dried Tomato Pâté/Dip

Serves 4

Ingredients

1 medium aubergine

1 heaped tbsp. light tahini

5-6 large sun-dried tomatoes, chopped

1 clove garlic, chopped

2 tsp. olive oil

1 tsp. fresh chives, chopped

1 tsp. fresh thyme, chopped

salt and pepper to taste

Directions

1. Wrap the aubergine in foil paper and bake in a medium heat oven for 1 hour or until soft. Allow to cool, then cut into chunks.
2. Put aubergine, sun-dried tomatoes, garlic, olive oil, tahini and fresh herbs into a food processor and blend until smooth.
3. Put mixture into a pan, heat through for 10 minutes and season to taste.

White Bean Purée

Serves 2-4 as a side

Ingredients

1 tin black-eyed peas, cooked, drained and rinsed well

2 garlic cloves, minced

2 tbsp. fresh parsley, chopped

1 tsp. cumin powder

1 tsp. chilli powder

2 tbsp. olive oil

150ml water, more if needed

2 tsp. Himalayan or sea salt

Directions

1. Place all ingredients into a food processor and blend until smooth.

2. Serve immediately or store in refrigerator.

Nut or Seed Butters

Ingredients

700g nuts or seeds, soaked (as per the soaking table earlier in this book) and dried

½ tsp. Himalayan or sea salt

2 tbsp. olive oil

Directions

1. Place nuts or seeds into a high-powered food processor.

2. Add salt and oil and blend for 15 minutes.

3. Stop blending occasionally to push all the extra nut/seed mix down around the edges of the blender and to allow the machine to cool a little.

4. After 15 minutes you'll end up with a nut butter to spread on crackers, breads or even on potatoes.

Hummus and Grated Carrot Paste

Serves 4-6

Ingredients

225g carrots

225g cooked chickpeas

3 tbsp. light tahini

2 spring onions

1 tbsp. olive oil

fresh herbs, to garnish

Directions

1. Grate carrots finely.
2. Put the remaining ingredients, except the fresh herbs, in a food processor and process until the mixture becomes silky smooth.
3. Add water if needed to ensure you get the desired texture.
4. Add the carrots to the hummus, mix thoroughly and garnish with fresh herbs. Serve with a small salad and/or gluten-free crackers.

Guacamole

Ingredients

½ red onion, finely chopped

1 tsp. finely chopped garlic

50-100g coarsely chopped tomato

2 large avocados, peeled, pitted, and cut into chunks

1 tsp. fresh lime juice

¼ tsp. cumin (optional)

salt and pepper to taste

Directions

1. Add the chopped onion, garlic and tomato to a bowl. Crush the avocados, squeeze the lime over the top and add the cumin.
2. Add salt and pepper and stir well, making sure the mixture gets a bit mushy.

Kidney Bean Hummus

Serves 4-6

Ingredients

1 can of kidney beans, rinsed and drained

1 tbsp. seed butter, like tannin

1 garlic clove, thinly diced

3 tbsp. olive oil

2 tbsp. lemon juice

Himalayan or sea salt and pepper to taste

paprika, to serve (optional)

olives, to serve (optional)

Directions

1. Put all the ingredients in a bowl or food processor and mix well, season to taste.

2. Transfer to serving bowl and sprinkle with paprika and chopped olives and serve.

Garlic Mayonnaise

Ingredients

1-2 cloves garlic, crushed

290g packet silken tofu

180ml filtered water

1 tsp. Dijon mustard

1 tsp. lemon or lime juice

30-50ml olive oil

salt and freshly ground black pepper

Directions

1. Add all the ingredients except the oil to a food processor and blend until smooth.
2. Add oil slowly until it is the right mayonnaise texture.
3. Season to taste and place in a refrigerator for 1-2 hours before serving.

Gravy

Ingredients

1½ tbsp. olive oil

½-1 white onion, chopped

1 small clove garlic, minced or grated

1 tbsp. gluten-free flour

300 – 400ml gluten-free vegetable stock

salt and pepper to taste

Directions

1. Add oil to a heated saucepan.

2. Add onion and cook through, add garlic and cook until lightly brown.

3. Stir in flour and then slowly add vegetable stock and stir until thickened (if you add the stock too quickly, you'll get lumps).

DESSERTS

Pineapple and Orange Cake

Serves 6-8

Ingredients

150g dried, pitted dates

peel of 1 orange

the juice of the same orange, plus filtered water to make up
to 200ml

125ml olive oil

30g ground almonds

60g rice flour

90g gluten-free flour

60g gram flour

1 tbsp. ground ginger

4 tsp. baking powder

3 medium eggs (beaten) or a vegan egg replacement

150g pineapple

80g raisins

Directions

1. Preheat oven to 170°C / 325°F / gas mark 3.
2. Finely chop dates and combine with grated orange peel in a pan.
3. Pour orange/water juice mixture into the same pan and heat
   until simmering.
4. When dates and orange peel are soft, remove from heat and
   add oil.
5. Put date mixture into a large bowl and slowly add the flours,
   ground almonds, ginger, baking powder and then the beaten
   eggs (or egg replacement).

6. Chop the pineapple into small chunks and add to the cake mixture, along with the raisins.

7. Grease a cake tin with a little olive oil, put cake mixture into the tin and bake in oven for 30 minutes.

8. Reduce heat to 140°C / 275°F / gas mark 1 and bake for a further 20 minutes.

9. Remove from oven and turn out onto a cooling rack.

10. Can be frozen if you want to save some for another day.

Apple Loaf

Serves 8 – 10

Ingredients

5 apples, grated

200g of almonds, ground into a flour (I use my blender to grind them down)

200g of dried fruits, like dates, figs, apricots etc.

4 tbsp. of hemp powder

1 tsp. of cinnamon, ground

1 pinch of sea salt, ground

Directions

1. Chop the dried fruit and add to blender with all the ingredients apart from the apple, and mix well

2. Pour into a bowl with the grated apple and mix well again

3. Pour mixture into two small loaf tins (makes for more even cooking all the way through) or one larger one and pat down well

4. Bake at 175°C / gas mark 4 for 50-60 minutes

5. Turn out of the loaf tin and allow to cool

Cinnamony Apples

Serves 4

Ingredients

4 medium / large apples (cooking apples work best, but any you have is great), chopped into small cubes

2-3 tsp. cinnamon (or nutmeg or mixed spice if you prefer)

6 dates, finely chopped

2-3 tbsp. of honey (optional)

6-8 tbsp. filtered water

Directions

1. Add the water, apples and cinnamon to a saucepan over a medium heat and allow to simmer.

2. Once the apple begins to soften, add the dates and honey

3. If apples are still not soft and water has evaporated, add a little more water.

4. Stir continuously.

5. Once everything is soft and cooked through, serve as is, or with cashew ice-cream, custard or cream.

Strawberry and Lime Sorbet

Serves 6

Ingredients

450g fresh strawberries, hulled (you can use other berries as well)

5-6 tbsp. fresh lime juice, to taste

50ml agave nectar

100ml filtered water

Directions

1. In a food processor, combine all ingredients and process until smooth. Adjust agave nectar or lime juice to taste.
2. Pour mixture into a sandwich box and place in your freezer for a few hours.
3. Scrape the mixture from the sides of the box with a fork and mix to break it up a little. Return to freezer. Remove and scrape every hour thereafter until the mixture has been in the freezer for 4-5 hours.
4. When it's firm enough, scrape into a bowl and serve.

Peach Crumble

Serves 4

Ingredients

6 large peaches, peeled and sliced (or other fruit if you prefer)

4 tbsp. chia seeds, soaked in water for 1 hour

2 tbsp. coconut sugar

1 tsp. cinnamon

2 tbsp. lemon juice

handful of oats

handful of mixed ground seeds (and/or nuts)

2 tbsp. honey (optional)

4 small ramekins

Directions

1. Preheat oven to 180°C / 350°F / gas mark 4.
2. Blend soaked chia seeds, coconut sugar, cinnamon, and lemon juice in a blender.
3. In a bowl, fold the blended chia seed mixture into the sliced peaches.
4. Divide the mixture evenly among the ramekins.
5. Sprinkle with oats and nut mixture over the fruit mixture in the ramekins and drizzle with honey if you wish.
6. Place the ramekins on a baking tray and bake in the oven for 30-40 minutes.
7. *Serve with dairy-free ice cream or custard.*

Choc Chip Cookies

Ingredients

90g almond meal

1 tbsp. coconut flour

1 tbsp. coconut oil

1 large egg

1 tsp. honey

½ tsp. vanilla extract

½ tsp. baking powder

2 tbsp. unsweetened almond milk

3 tbsp. dairy-free chocolate chips

Directions

1. Preheat oven to 180ºC / 350ºF / gas mark 4. Oil baking tray with coconut oil.
2. In a bowl, mix together almond meal, coconut flour, and baking powder. Then add all the wet ingredients and mix well.
3. Add in the chocolate chips and fold through the mixture.
4. Make 12 cookie shapes from the dough and place on the baking tray.
5. Bake for 8-10 minutes and then allow to cool to firm up.

Sweet Potato Cookies

Ingredients

380g gluten-free oat flour

½ tsp. cardamom

1 tsp. ground cinnamon

1 large sweet potato, roasted, peeled and mashed

120ml coconut oil, melted

180ml unsweetened coconut milk

2 tsp. vanilla extract

1 tsp. baking soda

¾ tsp. Himalayan salt

handful of dried fruits (optional)

1-2 tsp. honey (optional)

Directions

1. Preheat oven to 350°F / 180°C / gas mark 4. Oil a cookie sheet with a little coconut oil.

2. Mix together dry ingredients in a bowl. Add wet ingredients and mix well by hand or on slow speed of a food processor.

3. Make 10-12 cookie shapes out of batter and place on cookie sheets in the middle of the oven.

4. Bake for about 20-22 minutes until cookies are golden brown and crumbly. Transfer to a wire rack to cool.

Pumpkin Seed Oat Biscuits

Makes 18 biscuits

Ingredients

90g oat bran

30g pumpkin seeds

20g pumpkin seeds to be added separately

45g almond flour

55g coconut oil, melted

45g arrowroot powder

55g unsweetened almond milk

⅛ tsp. cayenne powder

½ tsp. dried thyme leaves

¼ tsp. Himalayan or sea salt

Directions

1. Preheat oven to 350°F/180°C/gas mark 6 and place some greaseproof paper on a baking tray.
2. Add the oat bran and the 30g of pumpkin seeds to a food processor and blend for no more than 30 seconds.
3. Now add the almond flour, arrowroot, salt, cayenne and thyme and just blend long enough so it's all well mixed.
4. Place all the blended ingredients in a large bowl and add the coconut oil. Rub mixture between your figures to make breadcrumbs.
5. Add the almond milk and mix together to form a dough.
6. Add the remaining pumpkin seeds.
7. Roll dough out between two pieces of greaseproof paper, until roughly ¼ inch thick and cut into biscuit shapes of your choosing.
8. Bake for 15 minutes. The biscuit edges should be golden, but not browned.
9. Allow to cool on a wire rack.

Coconut and Chocolate Macaroons

Makes 10 macaroons

Ingredients

300g desiccated coconut

60g warm water

60g coconut oil, melted

3 eggs, beaten

60g raw cacao powder, optional

2-3 tsp. alcohol free vanilla extract

Directions

1. Preheat oven to 350°F/180°C/gas mark 6 and place some greaseproof paper on a baking tray.

2. Place the coconut, warm water and melted oil and stir until mixed very well.

3. Whisk the eggs in a separate bowl and add to the coconut mixture and stir in well.

4. Add the vanilla and cacao powder to the mixture and stir well.

5. Place a dessert spoon full of mix onto the greaseproof paper at 3 inch intervals and bake for 15 minutes.

6. Allow to cool on a wire rack.

Chocolate Bites

Makes roughly 32 bites

Ingredients

325g coconut oil, melted

220g of any nut or seed butter

140g cacao powder

2 tsp. alcohol free vanilla extract

Directions

1. In a bowl, stir the coconut oil, nut butter, cacao powder and vanilla together until well mixed.
2. Pour into ice cube trays or small moulds and freeze for at least one hour.
3. Store in freezer and pop out the tray 10-15 minutes before needed.

Vegan Mince Pies

Makes: 16–18 Mince Pies

Pastry ingredients

400g almonds, ground

400g dates

4 tbsp. coconut oil

1 tbsp. vanilla extract (non-alcoholic)

2 tbsp. agave nectar

2 tbsp. water

Filling ingredients

2 apples, chopped into small pieces

50g apricots, chopped

100g raisins

50g sultanas

juice and zest of 3 oranges

2 tbsp. agave nectar

2 tbsp. of coconut oil

1 tsp. mixed spice, ground

2 tsp. cinnamon, ground

1 tsp. ginger, ground

1 tsp. vanilla extract

Directions

1. Preheat oven to 180°C / gas mark 4.
2. Place all the fruit with about 100ml of water into a pan and cook through until soft.
3. While the fruit is cooking, add all the pastry ingredients to a food processor and process until well blended.
4. Grease each section of a bun tin with a little melted coconut oil.
5. Flour your kitchen worktop and roll pastry out to around 0.5cm thick and cut out circles to fit your bun tin.

6. Place the pastry circles in the bun tin and put in the oven for 5 minutes (they will still appear moist when removed).

7. With the remaining pastry, cut out shapes for the top of the pies (I like hearts, but stars or circles work well also).

8. Add filling and place pastry on top (do not overfill).

9. Place in oven for 10-12 minutes.

10. Again, they will appear soft, but they will harden when they cool down.

UK Measurements	USA Measurements
240ml	1 cup
480ml	1 pint
950ml	1 quart
125g flour	1 cup flour
225g butter	1 cup butter
170g sugar	1 cup sugar
90g oats	1 cup uncooked oats
170g rice	1 cup uncooked rice
100g chopped nuts	1 cup chopped nuts
140g dried fruit	1 cup dried fruit

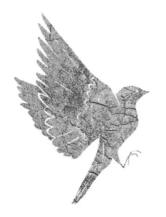

CHAPTER 12

A LESS TOXIC HOME

*Home is where one starts from – **T. S. Eliot***

Most of us realise that we need to detoxify our body and mind, but what about our homes?

What can we do to help reduce the toxic levels of our homes, apart from moving into a cave, tent or eco-build in the middle of nowhere? Well, plenty actually, and it doesn't have to cost a fortune either!

Most homes are full of toxic chemicals, which come from the building itself, furniture, paints, metals, carpets, fabrics, plastics and much more. These toxins seep into our bodies through direct skin contact, inhalation, or we ingest them through our food and drink.

Many of these toxins are hormone disrupters and can cause respiratory issues, asthma, tremors, behaviour issues, mild forms of depression, obesity issues, allergies, headaches, dizziness, fatigue and chemical and food sensitivities.

Older items can contain high levels of toxic chemicals. Mercury, for instance, was used in old clock pendulums, for the backing of mirrors, in the bases of some lamps and in barometers.

You don't have to throw these all out to create a less toxic home, but you do need to look at ways in which you can live more healthily with these items in your environment.

There are some really simple and easy steps you can take to do this:

- ❀ Stop using toxic cleaning products in your home. These are absorbed through the skin, through food that has come into contact with them, and we inhale them. They harm us and, then, of course, the environment, when they are washed down the plug hole (more about this later on in this book).

- ❀ Ditch the furniture, carpet and air fresheners. They do little to 'freshen' the air and actually are incredibly toxic for our bodies. Use a selection of essential oils and water in a spray bottle, an oil burner or simply sprinkle sodium bicarbonate (bi-carb) onto carpets and furniture, let sit and then vacuum up. Bi-carb is a brilliantly effective, safe and natural deodorizer.

- ❀ Open your windows as much as possible to let fresh air in and bad/toxic fumes out.

- ❀ Detox your body, hair, skin and four-legged friends (more about this later on in this book).

- ❀ Buy old, second-hand furniture where possible. This sort of furniture was generally made with fewer toxic chemicals (unless lead-based paint was used) and the chemicals that were used will for the most part have already off-gassed most of their toxic fumes. You'll also

be putting in a bid for reducing deforestation!! And you
may find that older furniture is nicer!

❀ Try to avoid buying furniture made of chipboard and
pressed woods. These are packed full of lots of toxic
chemicals, especially formaldehyde.

❀ Try to avoid furniture that has been glued together,
and opt for traditionally-made furniture in which glue is
usually not used.

❀ Avoid single-use plastics and soft flexible plastics,
like shower curtains, tablecloths and furniture covers.
These are full of toxic chemicals: some of the worst
are phthalates. Phthalates disrupt hormones and
are particularly bad for pregnant women and small
children as they impair child development. Vinyl,
especially, should be avoided at all costs as it's one of
the most toxic plastics around.

❀ If a new purchase has a strong smell, then put it
outside for a bit. Natural sunlight helps break down the
toxins that create the smell.

❀ Only use non-toxic (low VOC - volatile organic
compound) paints, waxes and varnishes in your home.

❀ Use natural fibre carpets and rugs.

❀ Try to avoid having clothes and furniture dry-cleaned
unless an eco-cleaner does it, as a whole host of toxic
chemicals are used by standard cleaners.

❀ Where possible, use and wear natural fibre fabrics.

- Avoid canned foods: the inside of the can (especially if damaged or if holding an acidic food) contains many toxic chemicals that leach into your food. Opt for glass or carton containers, or eat fresh, which is best.

- Avoid non-stick cookware. Go for ceramic where possible. Ceramic lasts almost forever, is easy to clean and won't leach aluminium and other toxins into your food.

- Dust and vacuum frequently, using only natural non-toxic products. This will remove chemical dust particles.

- This one can be a little pricey: invest in a home air filtration system. This will filter the air you breathe, removing toxic chemicals.

- Buy an under-the-sink water filtration system (these are actually fairly reasonably priced these days and easy to install). Invest in screw-in filters for all the remaining sinks and showers. This will minimise those pesky toxins in your standard tap water.

- Wash your clothes and fabrics in a natural washing powder or use soap nuts.

- Purchase as many detoxifying plants as possible. All plants detoxify to a degree, but some do a better job than others. Here are my top five detoxifying plants:

    - Snake Plant: filters benzene, formaldehyde, trichloroethylene, xylene and toluene.

    - Peace Lily: filters the same as above plus ammonia.

* Florist's Daisy: filters the same toxins as the Peace Lily.

* English Ivy: filters the same toxins as the Peace Lily.

* Aloe Vera: filters benzene and formaldehyde.

* You may think that burning a scented candle is better than spraying a toxic air-freshener, but I'm afraid that candles are just as bad: most candles are full of chemically-based scents and colourings and are also made of petroleum, making them very toxic. Either buy your own beeswax or soy (GMO-free) candles or make them at home (recipe for these later on in this book).

* Buy a Himalayan salt lamp or candleholders. Himalayan salt draws toxins out of its surrounding environment. It also ionises the air and will also draw dampness from the air. If you have a particularly damp home, then I would not recommend the lamp (it is electric and draws humidity towards it). Buy candleholders instead, and put these in a bowl to catch the water particles which will be drawn towards them.

Helpful Hints:

* A great rule of thumb: if you can smell it then you are also breathing it in.

* The more toxins are heated, the more they are leaching into the air. Try to keep all plastic and new furniture away from hot radiators or direct sunlight.

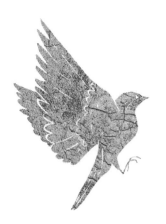

CHAPTER 13

LESS TOXIC BODY CARE PRODUCTS

Your body is a temple, but only if you treat it as one – **Astrid Alauda**

Toxins in our body, hair and dental care products are perhaps the most worrying of all the toxins discussed so far. I say this because it is believed that 60% of the products we put onto our skin are absorbed. The fact that the chemicals in the nicotine and contraceptive control patches we wear are absorbed straight into our blood stream only proves the accuracy of this claim. Unlike the food we eat, the products we apply on our skin do not get filtered by our digestive system. Instead, they enter straight into our lymphatic system and are carried around in our blood. They are also stored in our fatty tissues.

When you look at the ingredients in most of these products, you'll be hard pushed to understand what any of them are. The reason for this is because most are chemicals produced in a laboratory to enhance our looks in one way or another. The sad truth is that if we weren't laden with toxins in the first place, we probably wouldn't need these products to fill out lines, cover up eye-bags, deal with wrinkles and make skin 'look' healthier and younger.

Some of the many side effects of toxic overload are premature ageing, poor skin and hair health and reduced collagen levels. It's madness to add more toxins to make ourselves look younger to try to counteract the damage that already present toxins are doing to our beautiful bodies. If you detox body and mind, you will, by default, start to look and feel younger. Toxins actually age your body at a quicker rate instead of making you look more youthful. Some of the gurus of the health world look around twenty years younger than they are. This isn't because they have good genes, but because their toxic load is so much lower. The moral to this story: if you want to look younger, then reduce your toxic load!

One of the natural bodily functions of sweating is to eliminate toxins. Therefore, when we stop ourselves from sweating by using antiperspirants, we not only reduce our ability to eliminate toxins, but also put a host of additional chemicals into our bodies. If you start to reduce your toxic load in some of the other ways mentioned throughout this book, you will be surprised by how much less you sweat and that when you do sweat, it won't be anywhere near as smelly. Smelly sweat is toxic sweat - much better out than in!

Below is a list of some of the most common toxic ingredients in skin and hair care products and how they may affect overall health:

- **DEA/TEA/MEA:** suspected carcinogens used as foaming agents in shampoos, body washes, and soaps.
- **Formaldehyde:** suspected carcinogen and irritant in nail and false eyelash products, hair dye and shampoos.
- **Fragrance/perfume:** chemicals, such as phthalates. Connected to headaches, dizziness, asthma and allergies.

❀ **Mercury:** known to impair brain development. Found in mascara and some eye products.

❀ **Oxybenzone:** found in sunscreens. It is collected in fatty tissue and is linked to allergies, hormone disruption and cellular damage.

❀ **Parabens:** used as preservatives. Linked to cancer, endocrine and reproductive disruption. Some of the paraben groups you may find listed are: methyl, propyl, butyl and ethyl.

❀ **Imidazolidinyl** urea and diazolidinyl urea: These are the most commonly used preservatives after the parabens. May cause dermatitis.

❀ **Petrolatum**: in lip products. May cause skin photosensitivity (promotes sun damage), interferes with the body's own natural moisturising mechanism, and leads to dry and chapped skin.

❀ **Propylene Glycol**: ideally this is from natural ingredients, but it is usually found in its synthetic form in a petrochemical mix. Has been known to cause allergic reactions.

❀ **PVP/VA Copolymer:** a petroleum-based chemical used in hairsprays and other cosmetics. May cause or worsen respiratory issues.

❀ **Paraphenylenediamine (PPD):** used in hair products and dyes. Toxic to skin and the immune system.

❀ **Placental extract:** used in some skin and hair products and disrupts the endocrine system.

- **Silicone-derived emollients:** used to make a product feel soft, it is linked to cancer and skin irritation.

- **Sodium lauryl (ether) sulphate (SLS, SLES): degreaser**, now used to make soap foamy. This is a skin irritant.

- **Talc:** found in baby powder, eye shadow, blusher, deodorant and linked to ovarian cancer and respiratory problems.

- **Toluene:** used in nail and hair products. It is an immune and endocrine system disruptor and is suspected of hindering foetal development.

- **Triclosan:** found in antibacterial products, such as hand sanitizers and deodorants. Linked to cancer and hormonal problems.

- **Synthetic colours**: they are labelled FD&C or D&C, followed by a colour and a number. Synthetic colours are thought to be cancer-causing.

- **Synthetic Fragrances**: the synthetic fragrances used in cosmetics can have as many as 200 ingredients. These chemicals are believed to cause headaches, dizziness, rashes, hyperpigmentation, coughing, nausea and skin outbreaks.

- **Triethanolamine** (**TEA**): often used in cosmetics to adjust the pH level of the product. TEA is thought to cause allergic reactions, including eye problems and dryness of hair and skin.

I find there is a good rule of thumb when reading ingredients labels. If you have to have a degree in chemistry to read it then you probably don't want to be putting this product onto your body or into your hair.

Our bodies have an amazing capacity to deal with so many of the things we put on and in them. They eliminate thousands of potentially dangerous items from their systems every day. However, when we keep adding more and more toxins to our bodies, their amazing abilities become impaired and this is when the trouble starts.

I have read and heard many people say they believe that all of the ingredients in our skin and hair care products must be safe to use as they have been tested and approved for use. This is, for the most part, true. However, the problem is that these chemicals have been tested in amounts proportionate to the product they are being used in. So, if 0.001 ppm of DEA is used in a certain shampoo, scientists will test to see if that amount will have a detrimental effect on the user's health. What I've found out is that we use an average of 18 products per day. Many of these products contain the same or similar ingredients, and this is when that small amount of an ingredient that is thought to be safe, starts getting into our blood stream in much greater quantities.

The tests also do not account for the other hundreds, if not thousands, of toxins that are in our food, dental care and cleaning products and even in the air all around us. Once you factor all of this in, you will realise that as amazing as our bodies are, they simply cannot deal with these toxins.

Finally, most of these products have not been tested for long-term safety. Most of the tests and trials last for less than one month of continuous use, but how long do you use your favourite products for?

Dental Care

There are many toxins in our dental care products and we ingest and absorb many of them with a whole host of potential side effects.

There is a long list of the toxins present in all dental care products, including the ones used by your dentist and in items such as mouthwash and toothpaste. Quite often these toxins cause an imbalance in the ecosystem of the mouth and this then leads to tooth and gum problems.

The problem with fluoride

There is an ongoing debate these days about fluoride products and what they can potentially do to the body. While many dentists and health care professionals argue that fluoride is not only safe to consume, but it also helps our teeth and gums, this is based on out-dated information. Tests have shown that fluoride not only hinders tooth development, but also harms our overall health.

The fact that there are health warnings on most fluoride-based dental care products, that very few countries in the world now add it to their water supplies, and that even when taking some medications, you are told to avoid fluoride where possible, are just a few of the reasons I have chosen to discuss fluoride in this book.

Here are some of the side effects of consuming fluoride

- increased risk of thyroid disease (and worsening of symptoms if you already have this)

- decrease in bone strength

- acute body toxicity
- detrimental effect upon sleep
- may affect children's brain development and even intelligence
- arthritis
- hormonal issues
- kidney disease
- hypersensitivity (rashes, lesions, headaches, joint pain, fatigue, intolerances and vision problems)
- may hinder tooth development in children (yes, you read this correctly!)
- digestive issues
- infertility
- cancer
- cardiovascular issues
- hinders the absorption of antioxidants
- increased risk of Alzheimer's disease
- muscle pain
- hair loss
- weight gain

In my mind, this makes for pretty scary reading.

The Problem with Amalgam Fillings

Mercury (which is an ingredient in amalgam fillings) not only softens the mix so that it can fill the hole in your tooth, but it also helps to harden the filling, once in situ. It helps to kill bacteria that cause infection. However, there are a number of drawbacks to the mercury in amalgam fillings:

- Mercury is a highly toxic metal. It will leach from the filling into the body, slowly and over a very long period of time.

- Mercury can easily vaporise during chewing and could move up towards the brain. It is highly toxic for the brain and nervous system, and has been associated with autism, neuromuscular diseases, Attention Deficit Disorder and other nervous system conditions.

- Metal in the mouth can generate a flow of electrical current in this area, which in turn can affect the brain and general health of some people.

- Mercury can affect the immune system, the central nervous system, and the thyroid gland.

There are other metals in the filling such as silver, cadmium and copper and these can also be toxic to the human body. Some of the potential side effects of these are:

- diminished skin and hair health
- headaches
- fatigue
- depression
- brain fog, confusion and/or poor memory
- your toxic load is increased, and this can cause anything from weight gain to infertility

One of the strangest things about amalgam fillings is that any amalgam the dentist collects after your tooth has been filled is classed as toxic waste and must be disposed of as such. This is also true of any old amalgam filling which is removed from your mouth! How can it be classified as safe when it is in your body, and as toxic waste, when outside?

What you can do naturally to help

Firstly, you can swap your normal toothpastes and mouthwashes for more natural, shop-bought items or make your own very easily and cheaply. You can have amalgam fillings removed (by a qualified and experienced holistic dentist). And also, and perhaps most importantly, you can look at your diet! Ninety-nine per cent of dentists never ask what you eat or if you take supplements. With growing research that suggests a clear connection between dental health and nutrition, why is this?

Dr Weston Price, in his book *Nutrition and Physical Degeneration*, describes how he travelled the world, exploring the connection between healthy teeth and nutrition. What he found was that wherever refined food replaced native and natural foods, dental health quickly and severely declined.

Our teeth require many minerals that are missing from processed foods. These include zinc, copper, calcium, magnesium, phosphorus, manganese and boron. In addition, the sugar in our diet feeds bacteria in the mouth causing plaque. This opens the door to infection and can impair overall oral health. To top this off, our acidic diets damage tooth enamel and can even eliminate much-needed minerals from the body, causing additional health concerns. Good nutrition can not only prevent tooth decay, but can help the development of problems with gums and teeth.

The next section details my favourite replacements for toxic household products.

HOUSEHOLD PRODUCT RECIPES

Perfume Spray

Ingredients

one spray bottle

purified water

20-30 drops of essential oils of your choice

2 drops of a clear spirit such as vodka (not essential if you're likely to use this fairly quickly)

Directions

1. Fill bottle with water until almost full, leaving about 1 cm free at the top.
2. Add essential oils.
3. Add clear spirit.
4. Put top on and shake.
5. Shake well before each use.

Solid Perfume Sticks

Ingredients

2 tbsp. sweet almond oil

1 tbsp. apricot kernel oil

60g beeswax

¾ tsp. essential oils of your choice

Directions

1. Add everything except the beeswax to a glass bowl and place in a pan of boiling water.

2. Remove from heat and allow to cool slightly but not enough to harden. Stir in the essential oils and pour into small empty lip balm tubes or pots.

3. Put a lid on the container, once completely cooled.

Body Scrub/Bath Salts

Ingredients

¾ jar Epsom salt (for scrub) or Himalayan salts (bath salts only)

20-30 drops of essential oils of your choice

2 tsp. seaweed powder/granules (optional)

Directions

1. Put all ingredients into an airtight jar, put the top on and shake.

2. Use ½ cup in each bath.

3. Make sure contents do not get damp: keep top tightly closed between uses.

Place ½ cup of salts into the bath, allow to dissolve and then get in. Use a teaspoon of the salts on damp skin as a scrub.

Oatmeal Body Scrub

Ingredients

90g finely ground oatmeal

Essential oils: 8 drops lavender, 8 drops tangerine, 8 drops rosewood, 4 drops chamomile

1 tbsp. dried lavender petals (optional)

Directions

1. Add essential oils drop by drop to a Mason jar, stirring constantly to avoid clumping.
2. Application: combine one tbsp. of the mixture with a little water to form a paste; gently rub onto skin.
3. Wash off when you have finished exfoliating.
4. This will keep for up to 1 year in the fridge.

Vanilla Sugar Body Scrub

Ingredients

70g fine brown organic sugar

80ml sweet almond oil or other carrier oil

20 drops vanilla essential oil or 1 tsp. vanilla essence

Directions

1. Add vanilla essential oil to sugar in a Mason jar and stir thoroughly.

2. Add almond oil gradually, stirring continuously. Stop when the scrub reaches the consistency of moist sand.

Note: I also use a bamboo flannel. These are organic, natural, have no nasty colourings or chemicals and are slightly abrasive; they are a great alternative to body scrubs, especially if you have sensitive skin.

Bath Moisturisers

Ingredients

100g cocoa butter

20g almond oil

10g calendula oil

10g baobab oil

10g apricot kernel oil

20 drops of essential oils of your choice

Directions

1. Weigh out all ingredients.
2. Put cocoa butter in bowl and melt over a pan of boiling water.
3. Remove from heat, allow to cool slightly and stir in the remaining oils (including essential oil selection).
4. Pour into ice cube moulds and put in fridge to harden.
5. This will make approximately 24 small bath moisturisers.

Shea Butter Moisturiser

Ingredients

299g shea butter

50g virgin coconut oil

25g watermelon oil

24g avocado oil

1g vitamin E oil or grapeseed oil (this is your preservative)

20 drops of essential oils of your choice

Directions

1. Sterilise jars and weigh out ingredients.
2. Put shea butter and coconut oil into a glass bowl and melt over a saucepan of boiling water (don't overheat).
3. Remove from heat and add melon, avocado and vitamin E oils; mix well.
4. Add your chosen essential oils when cooled a little.
5. Put in the fridge for ten minutes before whipping. (This step cools the mixture further and helps with whipping.)
6. Stand the jug in a bowl of iced water and whip with either a hand or electric whisk until it has a creamy consistency. If using an electric whisk, do not let the mixture get too hot: this will prevent it from thickening.
7. Place the moisturiser directly into jars/tins; put the lids on and allow to set a little more.

Moisturising Lotion Bars

Ingredients

240g shea butter

240ml coconut oil

240g beeswax

10-20 drops essential oil(s) of your choice

3 drops rosemary essential oil to preserve

Directions

Break up the shea and coconut butter a little.

1. Place shea butter, coconut oil, and beeswax in glass bowl.
2. Place bowl into saucepan filled halfway with water (or use a double boiler). Place saucepan over medium heat.
3. Stir ingredients until they are all melted.
4. Remove from heat and allow to cool ever so slightly (you don't want the mixture to harden) and add essential oils.
5. Pour into your small soap moulds.

Note: I love both of the above moisturising recipes, but more often than not, I apply just coconut oil all over my body: my skin has never been better. Coconut oil also helps scars to heal, reduces itching and swelling of bites, stings and bruises, and helps heal them. All round, it's great for your skin... and a little goes a long way!

Hand Lotion

Ingredients

120ml sweet almond oil

60ml coconut oil

60g beeswax

1 tbsp. shea butter

1 tsp. vitamin E oil

10 drops essential oils of your choice

Directions

1. Put all ingredients except essential oils into a glass bowl.

2. Place bowl over a saucepan full of boiling water.

3. Allow the ingredients to melt. This can take around 20 minutes.

4. Once melted, remove from heat and allow mixture to cool a little but not enough to harden.

5. Add essential oils, if using, stir and pour into a jar. Close when hardened and cooled.

Shaving Cream

Ingredients

4 tbsp. shea butter

3 tbsp. coconut oil

2 tbsp. sweet almond oil

10-12 drops pure lavender or tea tree essential oil (optional)

Directions

1. Place a glass bowl over a pot of boiling water (a double boiler) and add the shea butter and coconut oil (breaking them up a bit whilst adding them) and let them melt, stirring occasionally.

2. Remove from heat once completely melted and allow to cool slightly but not enough to start the hardening process. Add almond oil and essential oil and stir to combine completely.

3. Transfer bowl to fridge and let the mix harden. Remove from fridge and use a stick blender to whip the mixture.

4. Transfer to an airtight container and use within a month.

Shampoo and Conditioner / Body Wash

Ingredients

1.5 tsp. guar gum

a selection of essential oils (totalling around 20 drops)

240ml filtered water

3/4 tsp. melted coconut oil

Directions

1. Choose the essential oils you would like to add to your conditioner. I like 5 drops of tea tree oil, 5 drops of lime oil and 10 drops of grapefruit essential oil. This makes a lovely, fresh, invigorating and anti-bacterial conditioner.

2. Weigh out and add all the above ingredients to a blender, mixer or even a smoothie maker. Add the water first before the other ingredients so that they don't have a chance to settle at the bottom.

3. Blend until there are no lumps (this takes less than one minute).

4. Transfer to your chosen bottle.

Note: You can also use just bi-carb for your shampoo and apple cider vinegar for your conditioner.

Anti-dandruff Hair Treatment

Ingredients

48ml jojoba oil

0.5ml vitamin E oil

25 drops tea tree oil

5 drops lavender oil

5 drops juniper oil

5 drops sage oil

Directions

1. Mix the jojoba and vitamin E oils together, add the essential oils and mix well.

2. Rub all the mixture all through your hair, covering the scalp well.

3. Cover with a plastic bag and then a towel and leave on hair for 10-12 hours.

4. Wash well with a natural shampoo, making sure to remove all oil.

Note: For damaged hair, massage either coconut oil, olive oil or honey into damp hair and let sit for 30 minutes. Then wash out thoroughly with a natural shampoo and conditioner.

Hair Spray

Ingredients

1.5 cups filtered or boiled water

2 tbsp. white sugar (add a little more, for more stiffness)

1 tbsp. of a white spirit (like vodka)

10-15 drops essential oil of choice (I like citrus oils)

1 tbsp. salt for more of a wavy beach look (optional)

Directions

1. Boil water, add sugar (and salt if using this) and dissolve completely.
2. Pour into a spray bottle, allow to cool, then add alcohol and essential oils.

Deodorant

Ingredients

2 tbsp. apple cider vinegar

25ml witch hazel extract

3 drops thyme essential oil

2 drops lemon essential oil

2 drops rosemary essential oil

2 drops either lavender or peppermint essential oils (optional)

Directions

3. Put all the ingredients into the spray bottle.

4. Shake well and spray underarms.

5. Shake well before each use.

Note: My favourite salt stone deodorant is by PitRock: it may seem expensive, but it usually lasts over a year, thus making it very economical indeed.

Cleanser

Ingredients

50ml filtered water

2 ½ tsp. witch hazel extract

4 drops lemon essential oil

4 drops juniper essential oil

Directions

1. Put all ingredients into your chosen bottle or jar and shake well to mix.

2. Put some of the mixture onto a cotton pad and apply to skin.

Note: You can substitute lavender essential oil for the juniper oil, but do not add both.

Face Wash

Ingredients

10 tbsp. grapeseed oil

10 drops lavender essential oil

5 drops geranium essential oil

5 drops rose essential oil

Directions

1. Add all oils to a bottle and shake gently.
2. Place a teaspoon of the mix in the palm of your hand and gently massage into your face, then wash off with warm water.
3. Store away from sunlight.

Note: Using oils on oily skin really helps to balance the skin's oil production.

All-Purpose Balm

Ingredients

Stage one:

14g beeswax

40g olive oil

18g jojoba oil

21g calendula oil

6g shea butter

Stage two:

12 drops vitamin E oil

20 drops essential oils of your choice

Directions

1. Sterilise your selected balm pots.
2. Weigh out all the stage one ingredients into a glass bowl.
3. Place the bowl over a saucepan of boiling water and melt ingredients.
4. Remove the saucepan from heat and whisk the mixture until it cools but is still runny.
5. Add stage two ingredients and mix well.
6. Pour into pots and cover.
7. Close pots when cool.

Once the procedure has become familiar, add any of the following essential oils to make a balm for a specific purpose:

Deep heat – lavender, ginger, eucalyptus and clove

Insect bite balm – lavender and chamomile

Cold sores – melissa, lavender and chamomile

Vapour rub for cold and cough symptoms – clove, eucalyptus, peppermint and chamomile

Mouth Wash

Ingredients

100ml water

100ml sage and/or chamomile-infused water instead of above water (optional)

1 tsp. baking soda

3 drops peppermint essential oil

3 drops of tea tree essential oil

1 drop myrrh or clove essential oil

Directions

1. Add all ingredients to your chosen bottle.

2. Shake well.

3. Swish around in mouth, and then spit out.

4. Store in a dark place, i.e., a bathroom cupboard.

Add 1 drop grapefruit seed extract, oregano oil or clove oil if you have inflamed gums.

Note: Another mouthwash I make up: I pick fresh sage and camomile from my garden, pop them in a large bowl and pour hot water over them. I let this steep for an hour or so, remove the herbs from the liquid, allow it to cool and then I bottle it. This keeps for weeks.

Teeth Cleaner

Ingredients

1 tsp. baking soda

1 drop thyme essential oil

1 drop peppermint essential oil

Directions

1. Put all the ingredients into a jar or pot.
2. Wet toothbrush with water, put it into the mixture and use as you would a normal toothpaste.
3. You may need to reapply half way through.
4. Mix up this recipe fresh, each time you want to use it.

Note: Oil pulling, (which is basically just gargling), with either coconut oil or sesame seed oil is a brilliant way to strengthen teeth and gums. Because these oils are antifungal, antibacterial and anti-inflammatory, they help with receding gums, mouth ulcers, bleeding gums, thrush of the mouth, general oral hygiene and detoxification.

Liquid Soap

Ingredients

200g coconut oil

200ml sunflower oil

100ml olive oil

180g filtered water

100g sodium hydroxide, also called lye (always wear protective gear when handling and using this, such as apron, gloves and eye protection)

10g potassium carbonate

10g grapeseed oil or vitamin E oil (these act as a preservative)

2.5ml of a selection of essential oils (I always use tea tree and lavender oils as they are antibacterial; I then usually add another oil, such as chamomile, ylang-ylang or a citrus oil.)

Directions

1. Weigh all the oils (except the essential oils) and put them into the small saucepan (pan 1).

2. Measure water and add to the bucket (or another saucepan (pan 2)).

3. Fill a large saucepan with water and bring to the boil (pan 3).

4. Put on all your protective gear. Weigh the potassium hydroxide/ lye and potassium carbonate and add to the bucket or pan 2.

5. Melt the oils in the small saucepan (pan 1) by placing in the large saucepan (pan 3) that is on the heat. Remove from heat when completely melted. Add the potassium hydroxide/ carbonate/water mixture in pan 2 to the melted oil mixture in pan 1 and stir with a long-handled spoon.

6. Now, stir mixture with a stick/hand blender until it comes to trace (this is when the stick blender makes patterns in the

Living a Life Less Toxic

thicker mixture as it moves through it).

7. Place the mixture back over the saucepan of boiling water (pan 3) and add a lid. Stir this mixture every 15 minutes. The mixture may look like it's separating or curdling, but this is fine. Make sure to keep topping up the water in the large saucepan on the heat as it will evaporate. You have to do this for 3 hours.

8. After 3 hours the mixture is ready to test for a safe pH level (which should be no less than a pH of 7). Remove a small amount of soap mixture with a spoon and place the pH strip on the mixture. Compare the colour it changes to with the pH chart that accompanies your pH strips.

9. You will now have created soap paste. Weigh 83g soap paste and dilute with 166ml boiling filtered water and dissolve well. If it does not dissolve, put back on heat until it does. Allow to cool down, add grapeseed oil or vitamin E oil and essential oils and pour into a 250ml soap dispenser using a funnel.

10. Put the remaining soap paste (if you have any left over) into an airtight container until you wish to refill your soap dispenser(s) and then repeat the last step.

Living a Life Less Toxic

297

Soap Bars

Ingredients

500g coconut oil

150g shea butter

350g olive oil

330g filtered water

154g sodium hydroxide/lye (never touch this without wearing protective gear such as apron, gloves and eye protection!)

3 medium figs (at Christmas I've used cranberries and cinnamon essential oil)

15ml honey

5ml grapeseed oil or vitamin E oil

15ml of a selection of essential oils (I like ylang-ylang, frankincense and jasmine – but this is completely up to you.)

Directions

1. Weigh out all the oils, putting grapeseed oil or vitamin E oil and essential oils aside.
2. Pour olive oil and coconut oil into one of the large saucepans. Cut up shea butter into small pieces and add to the oils. (It will melt more easily when the lye is added, later on.)
3. Put on all your protective gear (apron, gloves and eye protection).
4. Measure water and add to the other large saucepan.
5. Measure out sodium hydroxide (lye) and add to the water. Make sure you do this in a very well-ventilated area!
6. Stir the mixture with a long-handled spoon until the lye has completely dissolved.
7. Cut the stems off figs, cut into quarters and liquidise with stick blender.

8. Add fig liquid and honey to the lye and water mixture and stir until honey has dissolved.

9. Add the lye, water, honey and fig mixture to the oil mixture in the other saucepan and stir with long-handled spoon until all the oils have melted completely and become a liquid.

10. Now, begin to mix the mixture with the stick blender until it comes to trace (this means the stick blender leaves patterns in the mixture when moved around in it).

11. Add the grapeseed or vitamin E oil and your choice of essential oils at this stage and stir thoroughly into the mixture.

12. Put moulds (for making up to 1.5 kg of product) onto a tray. (I suggest this so that you can safely carry them.)

13. Pour the mixture into moulds and move to a safe place. Be very careful not to come into contact with the mixture yourself as the pH level of the soap mixture at this stage is highly acidic.

14. Allow the soap mixture to set for at least 48 hours (in some cases a day or two longer). It should set, but still be a little soft.

15. Wearing gloves, take the soap mixture out of the moulds. If you used a large soap mould then cut soap into individual portions at this stage.

16. Leave the soaps for a further six weeks to cure. Do not use them before this time without performing a pH test with pH strips. Simply place a pH strip on your soap and compare the colour it changes to against the pH strips accompanying the pH chart. You are aiming for a pH of 7 to ensure they are safe to use.

Sunscreen

Ingredients

120ml almond or olive oil

60ml coconut oil

60g beeswax

2 tbsp. zinc oxide (do not inhale the powder.)

1 tsp. red raspberry seed oil (optional)

1 tsp. carrot seed oil (optional)

1 tsp. vitamin E oil (optional)

2 tbsp. shea butter (optional)

Directions

1. Place all the ingredients except zinc oxide into a glass bowl and place the bowl into a saucepan of boiling water. Allow everything to melt down.
2. Remove from heat, allow to cool a little but not to harden and add the zinc oxide, stirring to make sure it's well incorporated.
3. Pour into a glass jar and allow to cool down totally before screwing on the lid.
4. Apply as you would regular sunscreen. Use within six months, and store away from sunlight.

Note: This sunscreen is not completely waterproof, and reapplication is needed after sweating or swimming.

Almond Oil – Sun Protection Factor (SPF) around 5

Coconut Oil - SPF 4-6

Shea Butter - SPF 4-6

Zinc Oxide - SPF 2-20 depending on how much is used

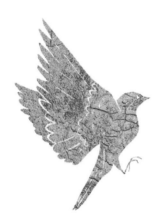

CHAPTER 14

LESS TOXIC HOMECARE PRODUCTS

*Water and air, the two essential fluids on which all life depends, have become global garbage cans – **Jacques Yves Cousteau***

We are often led to believe that we should disinfect every inch of our homes on a daily basis, so that we can stay healthy. This approach, however, does the exact opposite. Some contact with bad bacteria is necessary to build a strong immune system, and as infants, we need this contact so that early on, the body can recognise the bacteria as harmful and produce antibodies to it. If we never come into contact with bad bacteria as we're growing up, when we finally do in adulthood, it can make us extremely poorly as our bodies do not recognise them as harmful until it is too late.

When you add this to the negative response we have to the toxic chemicals in just about every 'normal' cleaning product you buy in the supermarket, this can make for some pretty poorly bodies.

Whilst many of the same ingredients listed in the previous chapter can also be found in our household cleaning products, there are others that you need to be aware of. They are listed below, accompanied by health issues they can cause.

- ❀ **Ammonia:** used in cleaning products. Irritation to eyes, respiratory issues, chest pains, burning and pulmonary oedema

- ❀ **Silica:** a fine dust, found in abrasive cleansers within the home. Carcinogenic.

- ❀ **Toluene:** used as a solvent in various products. Pregnant women should avoid products containing toluene as it is harmful to the foetus.

- ❀ **Trisodium nitrilotriacetate (NTA):** laundry detergent ingredient. Carcinogenic and also interferes with the elimination of metals in water treatment works.

- ❀ **Xylene**: an ingredient in stain removers, spray paints and adhesives. A suspected endocrine disruptor that can also cause memory loss through repeated exposure

- ❀ **Bleach (sodium hypochlorite)**: used in toilet cleaners. When it is mixed with ammonia, it can create chloramine gas. Both gases are extremely toxic to mammals and marine life.

- ❀ **Phosphates:** found in many laundry products (although this has been reduced). Also found at much higher levels in dishwasher detergents, which also contain high levels of chlorine-based (a form of bleach) ingredients.

HOME CARE PRODUCT RECIPES

Vinegar Antibacterial Spray

Ingredients

25 drops of essential oils of your choice

fresh water (to fill 2/3 of your chosen bottle)

white vinegar (to fill 1/3 of your chosen bottle)

half a lemon

Directions

1. Fill the kitchen spray bottle with 1/3 white vinegar and 2/3 filtered water.
2. Add up to 25 drops of a mixture of any of the following: tea tree, lavender, cedar wood, pine, lemon or orange essential oils.
3. Pour the juice of half a lemon into the bottle.
4. Shake well before each use.

I use this for cleaning my kitchen, all my windows and floors and almost everything else except wood. Be careful not to use it near or on any rubber seals around baths and sinks, etc., as it will eat away at these soft seals.

This recipe smells strong when you're using it, but the smell soon disappears once dried.

You can also use the peel and leftovers of any citrus fruit by adding them to the mixture. Leave the peel in the mixture for a week or so and then strain peel off (saving the liquid) and use.

Natural Bleach

Ingredients

fresh water (to fill ¾ of your chosen bottle)

1 lemon

hydrogen peroxide (to fill almost ¼ of your chosen bottle)

Directions

1. Fill an old kitchen cleaner spray bottle ¾ full with filtered water.

2. Then fill the bottle almost to the top with hydrogen peroxide and lastly add the juice of a whole lemon.

3. Shake well before each use and spray where needed like normal bleach.

Note: You can also use this in your washing machine (add 100-150ml per load) or as a soak for turning your greys white again.

Toilet Cleaner

Ingredients

240ml distilled white vinegar

20-30 drops tea tree essential oil

50g bi-carbonate of soda

Directions

1. Combine vinegar and essential oil in a small spray bottle.
2. Spray this mixture inside bowl and around the toilet seat and allow to sit for several minutes.
3. Sprinkle bi-carb around the sides of the toilet bowl and scrub with a toilet brush.
4. Flush toilet when done.

Bi-carb Deodoriser

Ingredients

Bi-carb of soda to fill your chosen receptacle

25/30 drops of your chosen essential oils

Directions

1. Fill up your chosen container with bi-carb (leaving about 2 inches of space at the top).
2. Then add 25/30 drops of a mixture of essential oils and give it a really good shake.
3. Sprinkle carpets and rugs, leave for a few hours or overnight and then vacuum it up.

This is a great carpet or fabric deodoriser, and it works wonders with eliminating pet smells!

Laundry Liquid

Ingredients

50g of a bar of soap (or save the last bits from used-up soap bars), grated

2 litres water

100g borax substitute (it is actually called this and you can pick it up in most supermarkets)

100g soda crystals (you can pick this up in most supermarkets)

100ml white vinegar

30/40 drops of essential oils (antibacterial oils such as lavender and tea tree work well, as do any of the citrus oils)

Directions

1. Pour half the water (1 litre) into a saucepan, bring to the boil and then turn down to simmer.
2. Add the grated soap and allow to dissolve (stirring occasionally).
3. Add the borax substitute and soda crystals and stir again until dissolved.
4. Take off the heat and add the remaining litre of water, then the vinegar and stir well.
5. Add your selection of essential oils.
6. Pour the mixture into any old glass or plastic bottles using a funnel. Make sure to leave an inch or so at the top of the bottle so you can shake it before each use (it will separate when standing for a while).
7. Allow to cool and then pop the lid on.
8. This laundry liquid can be used inside the drum or in the drawer and you will need approximately 50ml per wash.
9. You'll end up with around 2.2 litres of laundry liquid when following this recipe or you can double or even triple the ingredients to make more, as I do.

Note: I also use soap nuts. These are completely biodegradable; they don't come in lots of nasty packaging and if you order in bulk, they have a low carbon footprint. They are also really cheap. A 1kg bag lasts me about 14/15 months: each set of nuts can be used for around 6 or 7 washes, which means you spend £10.00 on soap nuts every 14/15 months!

Fabric Softener

Ingredients

200g Epsom salt or coarse sea salt

20-30 drops of essential oils of your choice

50g baking soda

Directions

1. Place all items in an airtight container and shake well.

2. Add 2-3 tsbp. of the mixture to your washing.

Note: You can also put about 10 drops of essential oils on a flannel: this is a good substitute for tumble dryer sheets. And to help whiten greys, add some white vinegar and bi-carb to your load.

Washing-Up Liquid

Ingredients

800ml boiling water

1 tbsp. white vinegar

1 tbsp. soda crystals

1 tbsp. grated natural soap

8 drops of lavender oil

juice of half a lemon

Directions

1. Pour boiling water into the bowl, add all the other ingredients and mix well.
2. Allow to cool and then pour into the bottle. Proceed as you normally do.

Helpful Hint:

There's not much that bi-carb and white vinegar can't clean in your home, so if you take nothing else from this chapter, I would highly recommend investing in these two very cheap and natural cleaners.

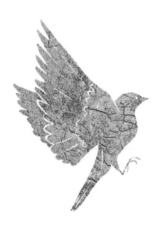

CHAPTER 15

DETOXING OUR FOUR-LEGGED FRIENDS

Outside of a dog, a book is a man's best friend. Inside of a dog it's too dark to read – **Groucho Marx**

You and your home are not the only things that you may want to think about detoxing. Consider your four-legged friends: both cats and dogs carry around a lot of toxins if we allow it.

In healthy animal bodies, toxins are rounded up and eliminated in more or less the same way as they are in humans, i.e. by and through the liver, kidneys, lungs, intestines, and skin. And, similarly to ours, our pets' bodies used to be very efficient at removing toxins from their system, but just like us, there are simply far too many toxins in standard modern-day homes for our pets to eliminate them effectively. Because their immune systems are on overdrive as they try to eliminate these toxins, inflammation and mucus production rates increase and diarrhoea can become more frequent.

The similarities continue, for when our pets are overwhelmed with too many toxins, their bodies are forced to store them until an opportunity presents itself to eliminate them. And if more toxins are added to their bodies, that 'opportunity' never arrives, and toxins start to accumulate indefinitely.

Animals can have just as many health issues related to toxic overload as their humans. Dogs and cats come into contact with a lot of toxins through their shampoos, flea, tick and worming treatments, when out on walks, from pesticides that have been sprayed in your garden or on surrounding fields, through their food and drinking water and, if they roam freely, through what they find to eat as they roam. They are particularly susceptible if they are already unwell, are very young or are ageing. Some of the side effects of toxic overload in your pets could be fatigue, vulnerability to infection, stomach upset, a weakened immune system, reduced appetite, early onset of arthritis and other inflammatory conditions. Abnormalities such as tumours and cysts may form, and other serious health conditions may develop.

Animals' bodies, again much like our own, are remarkably well-equipped to handle disease, eliminate a reasonable amount of toxins, and restore their own organs and body systems to health with some additional help and TLC. This includes, as a regular feature of their daily lives, a naturally healthy diet, rest, exercise and happiness.

The good news is that it's quite easy to reduce the toxins your pets come into contact with, especially around the home and garden. This will mean fewer toxins and better health for both you and them. This can be done by addressing all of the following recommendations:

- Reduce the use of toxic cleaning products, as addressed in the previous chapter, especially in the areas your pets are allowed. These products often affect pets in much the same way as they affect us, and sometimes even more severely.

- ❀ Improve the air quality in your home. Dogs and cats can passive smoke just as humans can. They can also ingest toxic air fresheners, perfumes and household sprays, so either eliminate these altogether or use away from your pets.

- ❀ Remove toxic gardening chemicals. If you cannot remove them from the entire garden, then do so at least from the areas of the garden your pets frequent.

- ❀ Make sure your animals are not nearby when you are cleaning your car, topping up the oil or washer fluid if you use toxic chemicals to do so.

- ❀ Try to avoid taking your dogs on any paths/roads that may have been treated with de-icer as this is incredibly toxic to animals, especially if they lick their paws, as most do.

- ❀ Regularly wash dog or cat bedding, using natural washing powder or soap nuts to eliminate a build-up of toxins on the bedding and to prevent more toxins from coming into contact with them from normal toxic washing powder.

- ❀ Wash your pets regularly (where possible, as I know they don't like it) to eliminate the build-up of toxins on their coats and paws.

- ❀ Use a natural pet shampoo or make your own (see recipe in this chapter), as normal pet shampoos have just as many toxic chemicals in them as human shampoos do. This is made worse for animals by the fact that they lick a good deal of these products off their coats after they've been washed.

☙ Regularly brush your pets. This helps stimulate the elimination of toxins through the skin and of course brushes away any toxins that have settled in the fur.

☙ Look at what you are feeding your pets. Most standard pet food is full of toxins, inflammation-creating ingredients that may lead to many health issues further down the line, and, to top it off, the food itself is not very nutrient-dense. Look for non-wheat-based foods and don't buy canned food if you can help it. If you are feeding your pets standard shop-bought foods and treats, you are undoubtedly giving them a dose of chemical additives and artificial colours and flavours with every bite. There are many natural and healthier alternatives to standard shop-bought products out there these days: take a look around and find one that suits you and your pets.

☙ Make sure your pet has fresh, clean (and preferably filtered) water whenever possible. Just as for humans, water helps pets detox and if it's good, fresh water, then you are putting fewer toxins into their bodies. There are more toxic chemicals in your pets' food and drink than in most forms of pet medication.

☙ Just like us, your pet's digestive system can be helped by a little of the fermented foods and drinks. I often add some of my surplus kefir grains to my dogs' food (just a few grains from time to time, however). This should help with tummy upsets, inflammation concerns, strengthen the immune system and support general good health.

❀ Pets, especially dogs and cats, can greatly benefit from greens supplementation (seaweed and green algae, etc.), just as we do. Most standard diets either have none of this, or very little. This will add a wide variety of nutrients to their food, including full spectrum amino acids, chlorophyll, antioxidants, trace minerals, and essential fatty acids. These will support overall health, flexibility and joint health, the digestive system and many of their organs.

❀ Make sure your pets get daily exercise, even if they are small. Dogs should be walked daily, rodents should have some form of exercise wheel or tunnels to play in and cats should be let out or played with daily. Exercise helps them eliminate toxins through sweat, remove mucus build-up from the respiratory system and keeps them fit and healthy.

❀ Make sure your pets are having daily if not twice-daily bowel movements. This is a key way for them to expel toxins from their systems.

❀ Although there is, of course, a need for medical intervention for yearly inoculations and medication as and when needed for illnesses, consider how much of the other products you need and how often. I find my

dogs are fine with one flea, tick and worming treatment
a year (just before the flea/tick season). Over the rest
of the year, I use natural flea and tick treatments,
(recipes in this book), and the fermented kefir grains
I add to their food prevent parasites such as worms.
If you do not want to make these treatments yourself,
you can now buy natural versions of all of them, either
from most veterinary practices or online.

❀ If you feel your pet may have some toxic thought
processes, brought about by previous owners or
traumatic events that may have happened to them,
then consider going to see a flower remedy practitioner
or a homeopath. They can suggest some natural,
healthy and easy-to-use remedies to help with
everything from separation anxiety to picky eating and
travel sickness.

Dog and Cat Shampoo

Ingredients

Reuse an old bottle (shampoo or ketchup bottles that you can squeeze work best)

1.5 tsp guar gum

a selection of essential oils (totalling around 20 drops) tea-tree and lavender work well for dogs and just lavender for cats (note – never use these undiluted on your pets)

100ml apple cider vinegar

100ml filtered water

¾ tsp. melted coconut oil

Directions

3. Choose the essential oils you would like to add to your shampoo.

4. Weigh out and put all the above ingredients into a blender, mixer or even a smoothie maker. Make sure to add the water first, so that the other ingredients don't have a chance to settle at the bottom.

5. Blend until there are no lumps (this takes less than one minute).

6. Transfer to your chosen bottle.

Cat and Dog Tick, Flea and Mosquito Spray

Ingredients

Reuse an old spray bottle

200ml water

400ml organic apple cider vinegar

2 tbsp. sweet almond oil

Plus:

For dogs: 2 tbsp. freshly squeezed lemon juice or 5 drops of lavender and 5 drops of rosemary essential oils

For cats: 5 drops of lavender and 5 drops of rosemary essential oils

Directions

1. Place all the ingredients in the spray bottle and shake well.

2. Spray liberally on fur/skin and leave to soak in.

Natural Deworming for Cats and Dogs

Grapefruit Seed Extract

This contains active ingredients that are anti-microbial, anti-fungal, anti-bacterial, anti-inflammatory and more. Grapefruit seed extract is known for treating over 800 strains of bacteria, viruses, over 100 strains of fungi, multiple types of parasites and it helps strengthen the immune system.

This a strong, natural anti-fungal/parasite, which should not be used long-term and only used within the guidelines of the label. The pet must be given plenty of fresh water and it is not recommended for kittens or puppies.

Natural, Anti-inflammatory Dog and Cat Treats

Use the left over pulp from juicing vegetables and fruit (not grapes though). Add coconut oil, around 1 tsp. per 200g of pulp and add 100g of fresh or tinned fish or meat and one medium sweet potato, cooked. Mix these ingredients together well and roll into small balls or long, fat sticks and cook for round 20 minutes in a medium oven (around 180°C) or until highly browned.

This is a great use-up recipe and will keep in an airtight container for around one week. You can also make these in a dehydrator and dehydrate for around 24 hours. These will keep for a few weeks in an airtight container.

You can also make meat jerky in your dehydrator for snacks or treats for your dog.

Natural, Anti-inflammatory Dog and Cat Food

I would recommend buying a brand such as Burns, Eden or another similar brand that do not use wheat or white potatoes, white flours or rice and do not add preservatives, additives or colourings. However, you can easily make your own dog/cat food by mixing a combination of sweet potatoes, fresh fish and/or brown rice and some root vegetables, and serve this to your pets. It is also advised to make up some dried food like the treat mix above, as the abrasive nature of this food helps to support good teeth and gums.

Helpful Hints

Many standard dog and cat treats can cause inflammation in our beloved pets. To avoid this, check the labels and avoid any with white potatoes, white rice and white flours. I add coconut oil, apple cider vinegar, rooibos tea, parsley water and kefir grains regularly to our dogs' food: these all help eliminate fungus and parasites from the digestive system.

Resources

www.ottawavalleydogwhisperer.co.uk

*The Complete Guide to Holistic Cat Care - **Dr. Jean Hofve***

*The Nature of Animal Healing - **Martin Goldstein***

*Complete Guide to Natural Health for Dogs & Cats - **Richard Pitcairn and Susan Hubble Pitcairn***

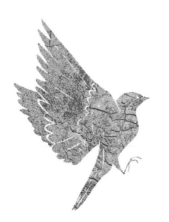

CHAPTER 16

DE-JUNKING HOME, HEALTH & OFFICE

*The first step in crafting the life you want is to get rid of everything you don't – **Joshua Becker***

You may be surprised to see that part of the whole life approach to *Living a Life Less Toxic* is about living a life less cluttered. There are a number of different reasons for including this in this book. Generally speaking, if you are living in clutter you are also living in the past.

Quite often, living in clutter implies holding onto things that have little meaning to your current situation, and not wanting to let go at the same time. This can lead to an inability to move on with your life, and that implies that you give inanimate objects more importance than they deserve or more importance than you give yourself. It can also lead to dwelling on the 'could haves, should haves and never will bes'.

If you are living in clutter you are most likely living in a mess, both internally and externally. When you look around you and see lots of 'stuff', you may find it increasingly difficult to relax, take time out and love being in your own home and space. You may become anxious in your own surroundings, you may not want to go home, or you may be tempted to live in only a small area of your home.

How do we end up with all this 'stuff' in the first place?

Marketers are very clever these days. They are not just selling us a single item: they are trying to sell us a way of life. They spend a considerable amount of time and money explaining that when you own this, that or the other thing, you'll be happier, your life will be easier, and you will never want for anything else ever again, that is, until the newer, better version comes out...

As many of us live in a state of general unhappiness, we equate buying new things to buying into a little happiness. For a short time, this is often correct. When we focus our attention on something we want, our brain's pleasure centre starts to fire and we produce more dopamine. When we have that new dress, new laptop or new car, we are often happy, flooded with dopamine, excited and proud of what we have. But how long does this really last? How long until you are saying to yourself, 'Oh, now I can save for this, soon I'll be able to get that', or, 'This would look amazing with that jacket, bag or those shoes I saw the other day.'

For most of us, I would say that happy feeling we got when we first made that purchase doesn't last much past a day, let alone a week, and then we are already thinking about the next thing that will make us happy. And thoughts of this next thing now flood our body with dopamine. The funny thing is, just the thoughts alone do the flooding: we never actually have to own that new item to have the brain produce this extra feel-good reaction in our body; we have simply to think about it. However, most of us are not aware of this. Either way, our brains are playing right into the hands of those pesky marketers. We start to measure our own self-worth on the items we own, the way we look and what our house looks like. The marketers want this; they want you to keep buying, they need you to keep spending, to keeping funding their businesses. That's the way the whole system is meant to work... in their favour, not yours!

We are caught in the marketers' web; it's hard to see a way out, without clinging to the next item we set our sights on. But that item isn't going to help you out of the web: instead, you're drawn deeper into it. So, how do you get out of this web? The first step is to learn to see that your self-worth is not based on the things you have, the people you socialize with or the places you visit. Instead, see how worthy you are, and what an amazing person you are, from the inside out.

How to improve the way you value yourself

3. EFT/Tapping is especially helpful with this. Tap on how you are feeling about yourself and how you think others feel about you and go from there.

4. Instead of focusing on the things you want, focus on how you would like to feel. So if you would like to feel happier, healthier, more energised, etc., then focus your attention on these feelings and make a plan about how you are going to make those feelings part of your life. When focusing on feelings, rather than things, you'll be happy and fulfilled with what's in front of you, and you will be investing in you rather than things. This kind of

happiness will last much longer than that new pair of shoes.

5. Start keeping a compliments journal (or add this to the back of another journal, book, or even list them in your phone). Whenever you start seeing your own worth in your possessions, you can refer to this and see that others don't see you this way - only you do.

6. Keep a journal or log of everything you have accomplished. Often we forget our day-to-day achievements and we focus on what we haven't got instead. The journal will help to show you how much you have actually achieved each day, week and year.

7. Get creative, get those feelings, thoughts and passions out, and into something that makes you feel good and also makes you feel like you are doing more than just your normal routine. You will get that dopamine flowing throughout your body, as well as other positive chemical reactions, and you'll have a sense of pride and accomplishment.

8. Stop comparing yourself to others. The grass is rarely greener on the other side and we all have our own battles. And remember: just because someone looks like they have it all, it doesn't mean they actually do.

9. When your inner critic starts speaking up, simply acknowledge it, thank it and then tap on it if it's still persistent.

10. Learn to accept yourself, know that you are an amazing

being, put on an amazing planet to be the best you can be. You were not put on the planet to be miserable, to compare yourself to others and just to buy the latest style in handbags.

11. Remember that what is really important is the health and happiness of the people you love (including yourself). Always wanting and pining over new belongings will never get you these two fundamental things.

12. Surround yourself with positive and supportive people, do not allow yourself to be put down, made to feel inferior or less than amazing.

13. Be yourself, be authentic. Don't try to be someone you are not: this will make you unhappy and exhausted.

14. As Dr Wayne Dyer puts it: "What other people think of you is none of your business." I know it's hard not to think about how others see you, but where does it really get you, apart from upset? Either they like you or they don't, and if they don't, they will leave, and if they do, they will stick around. Either way, that's their choice.

15. Treat yourself as you would want to be treated by others. By this I mean in a fair, loving, and compassionate way.

16. Look after yourself. If you don't, then who's going to look after everyone else?

17. Use loving, positive and uplifting visualisations and meditations daily. This will help flood the body with

positivity and love and create chemical reactions to reinforce this way of thinking and being.

18. Check out my book, *Loving Yourself Inside & Out* for lots more ways to love yourself and your life.

It's shocking to find you have become materialistic, which is what happened to me. I'm not sure how or when it happened. It crept up on me when I wasn't paying attention (that's sort of how it gets us all, when we are not present during our day-to-day activities).

I wasn't conscious of what was going on in my life. I didn't like myself very much and thought that I'd like me more, and other people would like me more, if I had a nice house, pretty clothes and all the rest that goes with these things. I never had much money, but the money I did have would be splashed at the next thing I thought would make me happy. And it always did make me happy on payday and perhaps for a day or two after that. But then I'd have that empty feeling inside; my bank account would be at zero again, and the whole process would start over.

However, once I started to practice some of the exercises from the earlier chapters of this book and from the list above, I slowly began to find that I was more authentic, truer to myself, and that I loved me for me and not for all the 'stuff'. The stuff just didn't matter anymore. And these days, the less I have, the happier I feel. I am actively trying to find ways to get rid of more stuff, free up more space and make money from all these items I thought I had to have, have barely used and never needed in the first place. I never set out to de-clutter my home this way. I simply understood I didn't like myself very much and this was hindering my health, both mentally and physically. And, holding on to all this stuff was leaving less room for the things that could and would serve me in my life instead. In fact, last year I sold my rather large home and all my possessions and moved into a campervan and have been travelling around the world ever since.

Why de-clutter?

* You will feel much more relaxed, happy and content in your own space instead of climbing the walls and wanting to run away from it all.

* De-cluttering your environment really does help to enhance many positive emotional and spiritual changes in your psyche. De-cluttering teaches you to let go of what you have been holding on to and move on.

* You will feel more balanced and calm.

* You should be able to sleep better.

* You will feel better equipped to deal with life on a day-to-day basis.

* You will have more time to pursue hobbies and get creative.

* Your general health may improve, and you will be subject to fewer illnesses.

* You will make space in your life, home, and most importantly, in your head, for new and exciting things.

* You will make money out of your clutter, or at the very least allow a charity to make money out of it when you donate it to them.

- ❀ You will be able to use your home fully, see and find important things easily and be grateful for the many wonderful things you have kept.

- ❀ You'll be able to return things you have borrowed.

- ❀ You won't have to go out to buy something again, just because you can't find it.

- ❀ Your allergies will most likely improve.

- ❀ You'll be more productive.

- ❀ And according to Feng Shui principles, you will have a healthier flow of energy throughout your home.

- ❀ You'll make room, mentally and physically for things that do serve you. For instance, if you de-clutter your home, you may find you now have space for that new person in your life. Or if you do the same in your office, you'll suddenly get new clients.

My top tips for de-cluttering

- ❀ If dealing with the whole lot scares you, just start on one thing, set yourself one task and do a little bit at a time. I recommend to clients they do a drawer a day. That drawer shouldn't take much more than 10 minutes, and we can all find 10 minutes in our day, right?

- ❀ Make a list of how you want to feel when you have completed your de-cluttering. Then write under each item a small task you could complete to help you get that feeling. When you are struggling with where to start or what to do, refer to the list and tick each item off as you achieve it.

❀ Always start with the easiest and simplest area first. This will help you get motivated and make you feel like you are already making progress, and it will enable you to move on to slightly harder areas next.

❀ Have three boxes always at the ready. Box one is for items to go to the charity shop, box two is for items destined for the tip or recycling centre and box three is for items that belong to someone else and need returning. If you have these always at the ready, then de-cluttering a drawer, cupboard or shelf a day is child's play.

❀ If you're a crafter, or know someone who is, then create another box for items that can be reused for crafting. However, make sure they are all in one box and are easy to find, otherwise, you'll never get round to using them for crafting and you'll find them in some drawer or cupboard and you'll have to de-clutter! Check out some of the projects in the previous chapter for ways to reuse your clutter.

❀ Give away an item a day for a year. This could be to friends and family, to charity, to the local school, church or playgroup or to someone who is homeless.

❀ Ask yourself why you are keeping each item. As Cheryl Richardson puts it in her book, The Art of Extreme Self-Care: Transform Your Life One Month at a Time: Is it useful, do you love it or does it serve a purpose? If not, why do you have it?

❀ If you haven't worn or used it in a year, why do you have it?

❀ Do you really need certain items to remind you of certain people or places, or is it actually all in beautiful memories in your mind? Or, if you do need the reminders, you could take photos of all these keepsakes, store the images on your computer under "Memories", and then bin the actual ticket stub, card or menu, etc.

❀ De-clutter as though you were moving to a new home soon. If you can't be bothered to pack it up and move it somewhere new, then why keep it now?

❀ If you haven't got it fixed in the last year, will you really ever?

❀ Create two piles of paperwork (or use boxes or drawers). Don't get caught reading each thing as you de-clutter (this wastes valuable de-cluttering time). Give the item a quick glance and put it in the 'to deal with' pile or the 'shred it' pile. Then, later on, when you are watching TV, for example, you can work your way through the piles properly and file or shred as needed.

How to stop the clutter from appearing again

❀ Instead of making that purchase, imagine your last holiday, your child's birth, cuddles with your pets, your wedding day or another significant, happy event or person. That same temporary feeling you would have got from that purchase, you now have for free from that memory. Do you really want that item? Will it really make you happier? If so, for how long?

❀ Congratulate yourself when you don't buy something, rather than when you do.

❀ Start to take note of how much money you are making on selling your clutter and how much more money you have from not buying more clutter.

❀ Make up an easy-to-use filing system, so you can file your paperwork as it comes in.

❀ Always have your three boxes (for charity, for recycling, for returning) at the ready, so you don't have to wait for a de-clutter session to put things to one side that you already know you are not using.

❀ Make gifts and crafts with your clutter so it gets a second lease of life, saves you money and so you can see the smile on someone's face when they realise you have spent time making them something instead of buying them something.

❀ Use old clothes for cleaning or as kitchen towels. Why pay for cloths to clean your house when you have old clothes you could put to use?

❀ Ask yourself if you really need the item, or is it just because (as my husband would put it) it's a new, pretty, shiny thing?

- ❀ Never buy a new item as soon as you see it. Have a walk round, go to other shops, even go home and sleep on it. If you really feel you need it after all this, then perhaps you do, but always give yourself time.

- ❀ Learn to love yourself. When you do this, you won't see your worth in your possessions and won't feel the need to keep buying more all the time.

Resources

The Art of Extreme Self-Care: Transform Your Life One Month at a Time - **Cheryl Richardson**

Banish Clutter Forever: How the Toothbrush Principle Will Change Your Life - **Sheila Chandra**

The Life-Changing Magic of Tidying: A simple, effective way to banish clutter forever - **Marie Kondo**

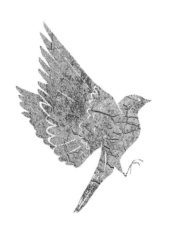

CHAPTER 17

NATURE NURTURES

*If we surrendered to earth's intelligence we could rise up rooted,
like trees –* **Rainer Maria Rilke**

Nature has the ability to heal us, but to what extent and how?

Many psychologists, therapists and doctors are now prescribing some time spent in nature. This can be anything from sitting in the garden to walking or taking up an outdoor sport. The theory behind this is that the stresses, strains, anxiety and even depression caused by modern-day 21st century living can be reduced or eliminated altogether with some time spent outdoors. Some people have even given this concept the name 'Eco Therapy', or as Richard Louv describes it in his book, The Last Child in the Woods, 'nature deficit disorder'.

Have you ever been for a walk in nature and felt ten times better afterwards? This isn't luck or just about taking time out from your day (although this does help). It's about our need as human beings to be connected to the planet, to reconnect with the healing powers of nature. When we spend days on end surrounded by electrical appliances, stress, non-natural lighting, recycled air and other 21st century norms, we disrupt our body's natural cycles.

This can cause a whole host of health issues:

- stress, anxiety and jitters
- depression and mood swings
- hormonal issues, including PMT and pregnancy problems
- ADD, learning difficulties and slow growth/ developmental rates
- fatigue, lack of concentration and brain fog
- obesity and eating disorders
- problems with eye development
- problems with feeling grounded and centred (feeling like your head is in the clouds)
- reduced creativity
- insomnia and restless sleep

There is now a growing body of research to show that nature is good for us and contact with it affects our overall mental and physical health. There have been many studies showing the positive improvements in people with mental health conditions when they spend time each day in nature. There has also been research to suggest that patients that were given access to nature in some way recovered from surgery more quickly than those that weren't. Our bodies function more effectively when we spend time in nature: we sleep better, we feel more grounded, we feel less stressed and anxious, and our muscles relax. Studies show that hormonal issues improve and blood pressure drops. Nature soothes and restores, we feel better overall and our body detoxes itself better. In the past, our relationship with our planet was different: we slept on the land, we worked it and it provided our food and drink. We no longer do this today. We actually spend very little time in contact with nature and yet we wonder why we feel so out of sync and poorly much of the time.

Electromagnetic stress

With this new technological age come new technological illnesses. Electromagnetic stress is the subtle, or not so subtle, effect of stray or chaotic electrical and magnetic fields on the human body. All electrical appliances give off electrical and magnetic fields when plugged in. We are also exposed to these fields when radio or microwave signals are received or emitted. These electromagnetic fields (EMF), much like our own body fields, vibrate constantly. When they come into contact with the human body field, they can disrupt cell structures, our immune, nervous and endocrine system responses, and increase the risk of tumour formation.

We spend so much time around electrical appliances and so little time in nature that more and more people are finding they are suffering from some form of electromagnetic stress.

Some of the common symptoms of nature deprivation are:

- ❀ colds, flu and general ill health
- ❀ problems concentrating
- ❀ anxiety, depression, aggression, irritability
- ❀ insomnia and general sleep problems
- ❀ memory loss and brain fog

- increased chance of (particularly epileptic) seizures
- dizziness, vertigo, disorientation
- fatigue
- worsening of already existing symptoms due to prolonged use of electrical appliances
- respiratory issues
- loss of appetite, over-eating and nausea
- high blood pressure and haemorrhage
- issues with the eyes in general but particularly in the cornea, and dry/itchy eyes
- eczema, dry, itchy skin, dermatitis and allergies
- joint and muscle pain
- tinnitus and other hearing difficulties
- low birth weight and foetal developmental issues
- persistent detox symptoms, burning sensations and sweating
- shaking and jitters
- developmental issues in children and adults alike
- vision issues, such as blurring and worsening eyesight
- not feeling grounded

The good news is that we can all make changes in our lives that will help reduce the effects that electrical appliances have on our overall health.

Here are some of my top tips:

- Remove as many electrical appliances from your

bedroom as possible, especially phones, laptops, tablets and TVs - actually, anything that is receiving or emitting signals of any sort.

※ Bin the electric blanket; these are possibly one of the worst items for increasing electromagnetic stress because they are so close to us for so many hours at a time.

※ Electric clocks, clock radios and baby monitors should be at least one metre away from you. (This distance will stop you from hitting the snooze button in the morning also.)

※ Switch off as many appliances at night as possible, and when you are not using them.

※ Do away with your microwave. Not only do microwaves break down most of the nutrients in your food, they are also a big source of electromagnetic stress.

※ Cordless phones are just as bad as mobile phones, so if you need to use these, then try to store them as far away from your body as possible when not in use.

※ Unplug yourself. By this I mean spend some time away from all appliances, in the garden, on a walk or at the beach, away from as many electrical appliances as possible.

※ Purchase a grounding mat or blanket for your bed. When you are sleeping, you will be grounding yourself. These earth through the normal plug sockets in your home. You can also pick up smaller ones to place on or under your desk to help when you are surrounded by office equipment.

❀ Try to avoid wearing rubber-soled shoes and slippers as much as possible, as you are unable to ground/ earth through these. You can actually buy earthing shoes, slippers and sandals these days, which help you earth as you are walking.

❀ Practice grounding meditations and visualisations.

❀ Consider wearing and/or placing all of the following crystals next to you or your bed or desk to help minimise the effects of electromagnetic stress: Smoky Quartz, Hematite, Tourmalated Quartz, Black Tourmaline, Amazonite, Sodalite and Unakite.

❀ Purchase a bio-band, a bio-tag, a grounding egg, earthing necklace or one of the other many grounding items you can carry around on your person all the time to help deflect the harmful effects of electromagnetic stress.

❀ Consider having amalgam fillings removed. They can make the effects of this type of stress even worse, because the metals in your mouth attract electromagnetic waves.

❀ If you can manage it, wear your metal-framed glasses as little as possible.

❀ Drink plenty of fresh, pure water as this has a wonderful grounding effect on the body.

❀ Use a Zapper, as I mentioned previously in Chapter

9. These not only help with many different health concerns, but they also help with grounding. This is because they emit a very low dose of negatively charged electricity, much the same as when the body is in contact with our negatively charged Earth.

❀ A Zapper helps deflect the positively charged electricity from our appliances.

❀ Ground/earth yourself. By this I mean go outside barefoot, with as much skin as possible touching the earth and spend some time connected with nature. Contact with the earth re-balances the body and brings us back to our natural rhythm and function. And this is my best tip as our natural state of being is to live, work, sleep and play in nature, and yet we simply don't do enough of this. I recommend at least 20 minutes a day of contact with the Earth to prevent many of the issues associated with electromagnetic stress. Paddling in the sea, hugging a tree (yes, hugging a tree) or gardening without gloves: all these are just as effective as wandering around barefoot for a bit.

A short note on Geographic Stress

Geographic stress is the harmful effect that earth radiation has on our bodies. Just as veins and arteries provide pathways for the transportation of our blood, the Earth has 'ley lines', which provide pathways for energy transmission around the globe. These energies are concentrated in certain areas, due to either natural or man-made phenomena. If you are spending much of your time at one of these concentrations, it can have a negative effect on your health. The symptoms are much the same as those of electromagnetic stress (see above) as it affects the body in much the same way.

Sometimes people find their children and pets sleeping in strange places, as they naturally try to move away from hot-spots of this type of stress within the home.

There are many people (dowsers, pendulum users, feng shui experts and intuitives) who can help you assess if your home is located over one of these areas. To help diminish the effects of geographic stress, you can use crystals, move beds and furniture to better and less stressful areas, use space harmonisers, pyramids, energy plates, geo-resonators, bio-bands, and bio-tags. See also many of the approaches in the section above.

Resources

The Last Child in the Woods - **Richard Louv**

Earthing – The Most Important Health Discovery Ever? - Clinton Ober, Stephen Sinatra and Martin Zucker

Toxic Childhood: How The Modern World Is Damaging Our Children And What We Can Do About It - **Sue Palmer**

The Stick Book: Loads of Things You Can Make or Do with a Stick - **Fiona Danks**

Run Wild: Outdoor Games and Adventures – **Fiona Danks**

www.earthinginstitute.net

www.kroschelfilms.com/grounded

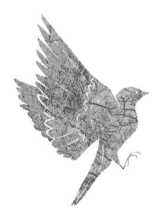

CHAPTER 18

WHEN BEING LESS TOXIC BECOMES TOXIC!

Not so long ago, I used toxic products on my body, in my home and in my car and garden. I, like everyone else, was brought up to think this was perfectly normal. I would have counted myself as someone environmentally conscious: I cared about the planet, respected nature, was vegetarian, cared about pollution, was a member of various nature groups and gave to various charities. I believed that if whatever items I needed were sold in my local shop, then they must be safe for me and the environment.

As I became ill and started looking into ways of getting myself well again, it soon became apparent that I was completely wrong in my assumption that these items were safe, and especially in the quantities we use them.

As I eliminated toxins from my body and mind, I started to feel better. I also realised I was spending far less money, enjoying making things, enjoying knowing I was helping the planet and loving the fact that the waste from our home had halved. When I clean my home now, I know that I am not ingesting toxic and potentially harmful fumes from the cleaning products I use. This also means these toxins are not getting on my skin or going down the toilet to pollute our beautiful planet.

However, as I started to become well from CFS/ME, insomnia, depression and IBS, I started to obsess about the toxins in everything around me. I started to think I couldn't go anywhere or do anything, not because I was so unwell anymore, but because of the toxic impact of those places.

I worried about the toxic effect of just about everything around me and my loved ones so much, it was causing me to become anxious and stressed out. I felt like I wasn't doing enough to reduce the toxic load of my home, environment and planet. I kept trying to do more, research more and change more.

Basically, I made being less toxic, toxic for myself. Because the stress and anxiety caused by this kind of thinking is incredibly bad, not just for mental health but for physical health also. As I mentioned previously in this book, our thoughts are super-powerful. If we are doing amazing things for ourselves physically, yet mentally thinking crappy things all the time, this has an effect on many areas of our health and lives. We won't absorb our food as well, or sleep as soundly, and our nervous system is on high alert and can then affect our digestive, endocrine and immune systems, as well as our mood and energy levels.

So, if your thoughts are anywhere near what mine were like, if you have made getting well, healthy, happy or even losing weight a stressful thing to do, then stop, take a breath and see how you can bring balance back into what you are doing. Stress, or just low level, long-term underlying overthinking will keep you exactly where you don't want to be. That's one of the reasons I believe it took me so long to recover my health, because I made getting well almost as stressful as all the years leading up to becoming unwell too. Doh!)

I'd like to make it really, really clear here. It's really difficult to maintain long term health, happiness and harmony if we only address the body and not the mind. If we only address the crappy food and not the crappy thoughts we'll only get so far. Or, we'll achieve our goals but then find ourselves right back at square one, some time later. I work with a lot of clients these days that recovered from a chronic illness in the past, only to find themselves relapsing a short time afterwards. There is always a common theme with these clients and that is that they only worked with the body and not the mind.

As I mentioned in more detail, in my previous book, *Loving Yourself Inside & Out*, the frame of mind you are in when you do something is almost more important than what you are actually doing. If you are eating healthy food but stressed with the calorie counting or making your recovery from a health condition really stressful, by constantly wondering if you are doing the right things at the right time, or if you are doing enough, then this level of stress/conflict will be having an impact on what you are trying to do. It will limit your body's ability to absorb nutrients, affect your immune system, energy levels, your sleep and even your hormones.

So, if you are getting nowhere, feeling stuck or are going backwards, how can you change your thinking about your situation? Try not to focus on the actual situation, just *how* you are thinking about it. You'll be surprised how quickly things change, but how they then stay that way too.

My dream is to one day see schools teaching students how to not only survive but thrive in the 21st century. I understand the need for doctors, bankers, politicians and business people, but our education system should also be teaching children the tools to deal with the high pressures they will meet in jobs like these, and even in living in society these days. Most of the clients I work with have been under high pressure for long periods of time, unaware there was another way - another way of being human, living in society and creating health, happiness and harmony.

Things could be very different if we were taught some additional tools at school or even in our working careers. If we could be taught to meditate, we could deal with stress and anxiety better, we could be more productive and sharper on the job. By learning gratitude, we could work better in a team, love our lives, enjoy the simple moments and suffer from less depressive thoughts.

By learning what foods to eat, where these foods come from and how to cook them, we would suffer from fewer illnesses, feel more energised, get more from our day and live longer and much healthier lives. By learning that stress and exhaustion is not an acceptable daily side effect of life, we would learn to listen out for the signs that our bodies are out of balance and address this balance before illness follows.

If we cannot or will not change what we are doing for ourselves, we simply must give our children the tools to help them manage their lives in a healthier way. With the increase in outside stresses, strains, toxins and potential hardships, we have a duty to care for the next generation to help them be a happier, healthier and more fulfilled generation than ours. This planet is a truly amazing place to live. Let's help the next generation see and embrace it, and themselves, in all our glory!